Musculoskeletal Imaging
A Core Review

Musculoskeletal Imaging
A Core Review

EDITORS

Paul J. Spicer, MD

Assistant Professor
Musculoskeletal and Women's Radiology
Department of Radiology
University of Kentucky
Lexington, Kentucky

Francesca Beaman, MD

Assistant Professor
Division Chief, Musculoskeletal Radiology
Director, Musculoskeletal Radiology Fellowship Program
Assistant Director, Radiology Residency Program
Department of Radiology
University of Kentucky
Lexington, Kentucky

Gustav A. Blomquist, MD

Assistant Professor
Musculoskeletal and Emergency Radiology
Department of Radiology
University of Kentucky
Lexington, Kentucky

Justin Montgomery, MD

Assistant Professor
Musculoskeletal Radiology
Department of Radiology
University of Kentucky
Lexington, Kentucky

Matthew E. Maxwell, MD

Fellow of Musculoskeletal Radiology
Department of Radiology
University of Kentucky
Lexington, Kentucky

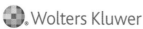
Wolters Kluwer
Health

Philadelphia • Baltimore • New York • London
Buenos Aires • Hong Kong • Sydney • Tokyo

Acquisitions Editor: Ryan Shaw
Product Development Editor: Amy G. Dinkel
Production Product Manager: Priscilla Crater
Senior Manufacturing Coordinator: Beth Welsh
Senior Marketing Manager: Dan Dressler
Senior Designer: Stephen Druding
Production Service: SPi Global

Printed in China

Library of Congress Cataloging-in-Publication Data

Musculoskeletal imaging (Spicer)

Musculoskeletal imaging : a core review / editors, Paul J. Spicer, Francesca Beaman, Gustav A. Blomquist, Justin Montgomery, Matthew E. Maxwell.

p. ; cm.

Includes bibliographical references and index.

ISBN 978-1-4511-9267-4 (alk. paper)

I. Spicer, Paul J., editor. II. Beaman, Francesca, editor. III. Blomquist, Gustav A., editor. IV. Montgomery, Justin, editor. V. Maxwell, Matthew E., editor. VI. Title.

[DNLM: 1. Musculoskeletal Diseases—diagnosis—Examination Questions. 2. Diagnostic Imaging—Examination Questions. 3. Musculoskeletal System—injuries—Examination Questions. WE 18.2]

RC925.7

616.7'075076—dc23

2014011385

Care has been taken to confirm the accuracy of the information presented and to describe generally accepted practices. However, the authors, editors, and publisher are not responsible for errors or omissions or for any consequences from application of the information in this book and make no warranty, expressed or implied, with respect to the currency, completeness, or accuracy of the contents of the publication. Application of the information in a particular situation remains the professional responsibility of the practitioner.

The authors, editors, and publisher have exerted every effort to ensure that drug selection and dosage set forth in this text are in accordance with current recommendations and practice at the time of publication. However, in view of ongoing research, changes in government regulations, and the constant flow of information relating to drug therapy and drug reactions, the reader is urged to check the package insert for each drug for any change in indications and dosage and for added warnings and precautions. This is particularly important when the recommended agent is a new or infrequently employed drug.

Some drugs and medical devices presented in the publication have Food and Drug Administration (FDA) clearance for limited use in restricted research settings. It is the responsibility of the health care provider to ascertain the FDA status of each drug or device planned for use in their clinical practice.

To purchase additional copies of this book, call our customer service department at (800) 638–3030 or fax orders to (301) 223–2320. International customers should call (301) 223–2300.

Visit Lippincott Williams & Wilkins on the Internet: at LWW.com. Lippincott Williams & Wilkins customer service representatives are available from 8:30 am to 6 pm, EST.

10 9 8 7 6 5 4 3 2 1

Thank you to my wife and daughter for their love and support. Thank you to my parents for teaching me the important things of life. Thank you to those who taught me at the University of Toledo and Henry Ford Hospital, particularly Marnix van Holsbeeck and Joseph Craig.

—PAUL J. SPICER

Thank you to my mentors, Mark Kransdorf, Laura Bancroft, Jeff Peterson, and Tom Berquist, for your instruction and encouragement.

—FRANCESCA BEAMAN

To my family, with whom I laugh, love, and labor.

—GUSTAV A. BLOMQUIST

To Kerri—thank you for your unending love and support. For Sullivan—who is deeply loved.

—JUSTIN MONTGOMERY

Thanks to Sara for your love and patience, and to all of my many teachers and mentors in Lexington.

—MATTHEW E. MAXWELL

Francesca Beaman, MD

Assistant Professor
Division Chief, Musculoskeletal Radiology
Director, Musculoskeletal Radiology Fellowship
  Program
Assistant Director, Radiology Residency Program
Department of Radiology
University of Kentucky
Lexington, Kentucky

Joseph M. Bestic, MD

Assistant Professor of Radiology
Mayo Clinic Florida
Jacksonville, Florida

Gustav A. Blomquist, MD

Assistant Professor
Musculoskeletal and Emergency Radiology
Department of Radiology
University of Kentucky
Lexington, Kentucky

Hillary W. Garner, MD

Assistant Professor of Radiology
Mayo Clinic Florida
Jacksonville, Florida

Peter A. Hardy, PhD

Assistant Professor
Division of Medical Physics
Department of Radiology
University of Kentucky
Lexington, Kentucky

Matthew E. Maxwell, MD

Fellow of Musculoskeletal Radiology
Department of Radiology
University of Kentucky
Lexington, Kentucky

Justin Montgomery, MD

Assistant Professor
Musculoskeletal Radiology
Department of Radiology
University of Kentucky
Lexington, Kentucky

Gopi K. Nallani, MD

Musculoskeletal Radiologist
Advanced Diagnostic Imaging
Saginaw, Michigan

Jay Prakash Patel, MD

Breast and Musculoskeletal Imaging Diagnostic
  Radiologist
Quantum Radiology
Marietta, Georgia

Jeffrey James Peterson, MD

Professor of Radiology
Mayo Clinic Florida
Jacksonville, Florida

Daniel Siegal, MD

Clinical Assistant Professor
Wayne State University School of Medicine
Senior Staff Radiologist
Department of Radiology
Musculoskeletal Division
Henry Ford Hospital and Health Network
Detroit, Michigan

Steven B. Soliman, DO, RMSK

Subspecialty Director
Musculoskeletal Radiology
Oakwood Hospital and Medical Center
Drs. Harris, Birkhill, Wang, Songe & Assoc. P.C.
Dearborn, Michigan

Paul J. Spicer, MD

Assistant Professor
Musculoskeletal and Women's Radiology
Department of Radiology
University of Kentucky
Lexington, Kentucky

William Wong, MD

Musculoskeletal Radiologist
Advanced Diagnostic Imaging
Saginaw, Michigan

Jie Zhang, PhD, DABR

Associate Professor
Chief, Division of Medical Physics
Department of Radiology
University of Kentucky
Lexington, Kentucky

SERIES FOREWORD

Musculoskeletal Imaging: A Core Review is the second book and the newest addition to the *Core Review Series*. Dr. Paul Spicer, Dr. Francesca Beaman, Dr. Gustav Blomquist, Dr. Justin Montgomery, and Dr. Matthew Maxwell have succeeded in presenting a very challenging topic in a manner that is straightforward and readily accessible to the reader. Part of the challenge in writing a multiple-choice question book on musculoskeletal radiology is the vast topic that it comprises in such areas of musculoskeletal trauma, infection, neoplasms, metabolic disorders, postoperative imaging, congenital abnormalities, arthritic pathology, and imaging techniques. They have divided the questions logically into different sections, as per *The ABR Core Examination Study Guide*, so as to make it easy for readers to work on particular topics as needed.

The authors of *Musculoskeletal Imaging: A Core Review* have succeeded in producing a book that exemplifies the philosophy and goals of The *Core Review Series*. Dr. Spicer and his colleagues have done a meticulous job in covering key topics and providing quality images. Each question has a corresponding answer with an explanation of not only why a particular answer choice is correct but also why the other answer choices are incorrect. There are references provided for each question for those who want to delve more deeply into a specific subject.

The intent of the *Core Review Series* is to provide the resident, fellow, or practicing physician a review of the important conceptual, factual, and practical aspects of a subject by providing approximately 300 multiple-choice questions, in a format similar to the ABR Core examination. The *Core Review Series* is not intended to be exhaustive but to provide material likely to be tested on the ABR Core exam and that would be required in clinical practice.

Dr. Paul Spicer, his co-authors, and contributors are to be congratulated on doing an outstanding job. I believe *Musculoskeletal Imaging: A Core Review* will serve as a useful resource for residents during their board preparation and a valuable reference for fellows and practicing radiologists.

Biren A. Shah, MD, FACR
Series Editor
Henry Ford Hospital

PREFACE

The changing of the Boards format has altered the way in which residents will prepare for the exam. Instead of hours of oral case review and interpretation, the preparations are now geared toward using images as a means to test residents' comprehensive understanding of disease processes, the physics behind image acquisition, quality control, and safety. The interaction with the oral examiners is in the past, and individuals are left alone facing a computer with multiple-choice and extended matching questions. There is a relative paucity of information and study resources available for residents, and we hope that this book will serve as a useful tool for residents on their road to becoming Board-certified radiologists and will continue to be a reference in their future careers.

Our goal with this book was to provide for residents a guide that will assess their knowledge and review the relevant material. The format was designed to be similar to the exam. The questions are divided into different sections to make it easy for the readers to work on particular topics as needed. Each question has a corresponding answer with an explanation of both why a particular option is correct and why the other options are incorrect. References are provided for each question for those wishing to delve more deeply into a specific subject. The format is also practical for radiologists preparing for Maintenance of Certification (MOC).

Multiple colleagues have contributed to this publication. The quality of this book, as well as its timely completion, could not have been brought to fruition without the efforts of all these wonderful individuals who took time from their busy lives to research, write, and submit material in a timely manner. To all who helped, we offer our heartfelt thanks.

Additionally, we would like to extend thanks to the staff at LWW for the gift of this opportunity and guiding us along the way.

Finally, we are truly grateful to our families, who have encouraged us through long hours of work and supported us each step along the way.

Paul J. Spicer, MD
Francesca Beaman, MD
Gustav A. Blomquist, MD
Justin Montgomery, MD
Matthew E. Maxwell, MD

ACKNOWLEDGMENTS

The authors would like to extend our heartfelt appreciation to Dr. Biren Shah for his guidance throughout this authorship process. We would like to thank the staff at Lippincott, Williams & Wilkins for allowing us to write this book and for making the process as seamless as possible. In particular, we would like to thank certain staff members at Lippincott for their help in this endeavor. These include the late Jonathan Pine, Ryan Shaw, Amy Dinkel, Priscilla Crater, Beth Welsh, Dan Dressler, and Stephen Druding. We would like to thank Sarah Granlund for her help with this project. We would finally like to thank Sree Vidya Dhanvanthri of SPi Global for her help and patience during the review process.

CONTENTS

1 Imaging Techniques/Physics/Quality and Safety

QUESTIONS

1 Which of the following MRI parameter changes would result in decreased
metallic susceptibility artifact?

Goal is to ↓ SNR

A. Increased receiver bandwidth
B. Increased field strength
C. Increased voxel size
D. Increased slice thickness

2a A patient presents for an arthrogram of the left shoulder. What is the preferred
needle placement for a rotator interval approach?

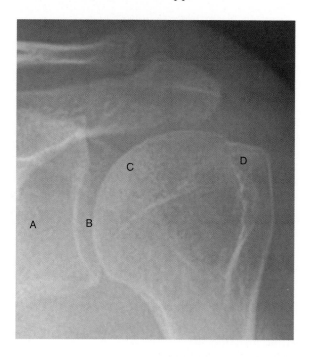

A. A
B. B
C. C
D. D

2b The patient is scheduled for an arthrogram followed by a CT examination of the left shoulder. What is the most appropriate mixture for the arthrogram?

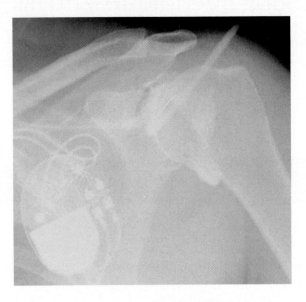

A. Iodinated contrast 1:1 saline and/or anesthetic
B. Iodinated contrast 1:10 saline and/or anesthetic
C. Iodinated contrast 1:100 saline and/or anesthetic
D. Iodinated contrast 1:1,000 saline and/or anesthetic

2c Which of the following is an appropriate reason for a CT arthrogram instead of MRI arthrogram?

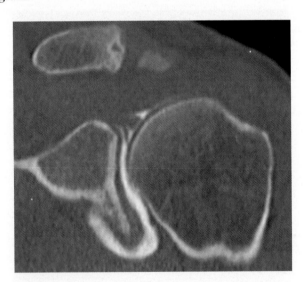

A. Lack of joint mobility
B. Anticoagulation
C. Infection at the injection site
D. Metallic hardware near the joint

3 Placing an MRI receiver coil farther than normal from the area of interest will result in

A. increased signal-to-noise ratio.
B. decreased receiver bandwidth.
C. decreased spatial resolution.
D. decreased signal-to-noise ratio.

4 You are called to evaluate a patient following inadvertent IV contrast infiltration. The technologist informs you that ~100 mL of iodinated contrast extravasated into the antecubital fossa. Which of the following is the primary clinical concern?

A. Compartment syndrome
B. Nephrogenic systemic fibrosis
C. Contrast-related renal dysfunction
D. Vasospasm

5 What percentage of bone mineralization must be lost to be detected by radiographs?

A. 10% to 20%
B. 30% to 40%
C. 50% to 60%
D. 70% to 80%

6a A patient presents for a left hip arthrogram. What is the preferred needle location to avoid complications with nerve, vessel, and bursa injections?

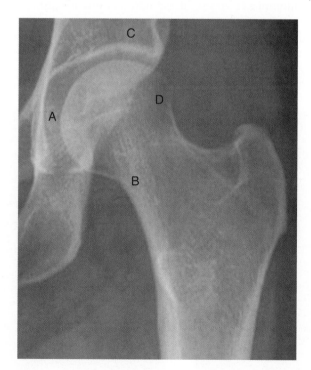

A. A
B. B
C. C
D. D

6b The patient is scheduled for an arthrogram followed by an MRI examination of the left hip. What is the appropriate mixture for the arthrogram?

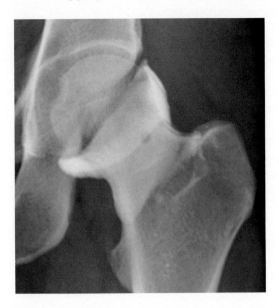

- A. 0.01 mL gadolinium per 20 mL of iodinated contrast, saline, and/or anesthetic mixture
- B. 0.1 mL gadolinium per 20 mL of iodinated contrast, saline, and/or anesthetic mixture
- C. 1 mL gadolinium per 20 mL of iodinated contrast, saline, and/or anesthetic mixture
- D. 10 mL gadolinium per 20 mL of iodinated contrast, saline, and/or anesthetic mixture

6c For which of the following scenarios is MRI preferred over CT after arthrography?

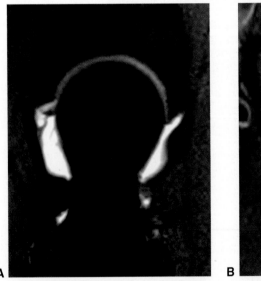 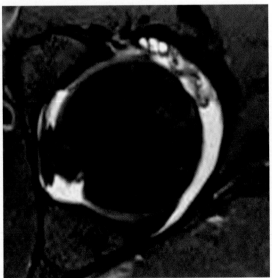

A. Sagittal oblique T1 weighted fat saturated **B.** Axial T2 weighted fat saturated

- A. Claustrophobic patient
- B. Potential cartilage defects
- C. Obese patients
- D. Prior labral surgery

7 The following image shows an artifact. From the list below select the best protocol change to eliminate this artifact.

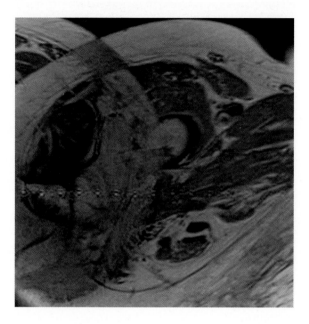

A. Double the image matrix.
B. Double the image oversampling in the phase-encoded direction.
C. Double the receiver bandwidth.
D. Double the FOV.

8 Fluid appears as increased signal on a T2-weighted image because it has which of the following?

A. Short T2 relaxation time
B. Short T1 relaxation time
C. Long T2 relaxation time
D. Long T1 relaxation time

9 Which of the following will achieve high-resolution imaging of small MSK structures?

A. Use 2D imaging with thin slices.
B. Use 3D imaging with thin slices.
C. Use 2D imaging with a large number of averages.
D. Use proton density imaging.

10 Which of the following would be the best method to achieve quality T2-weighted images in a patient with difficulty remaining still during imaging?

A. Use single-echo spin echo imaging.
B. Use gradient-echo imaging.
C. Use a radial imaging such as BLADE (MRI acronym, Siemens) or PROPELLOR (MRI acronym, GE).
D. Use the body coil instead of a surface coil.

11 What artifact is noted on the sagittal T2-weighted MR image below?

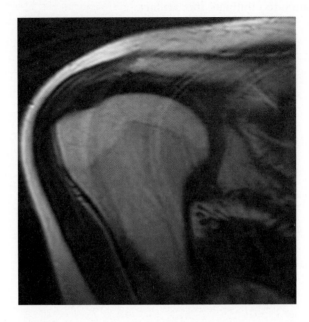

   A. Gibbs phenomenon
   B. Chemical shift
   C. Motion
   D. Wraparound

12 Injecting a gadolinium contrast agent causes a sarcoma to

   A. appear bright on T1-weighted images.
   B. appear dark on T2-weighted images.
   C. appear isointense to skeletal muscle on T1-weighted images.
   D. appear bright on proton density–weighted images.

13 Which of the following parameters can be altered without changing the total scan time?

   A. Number of excitations (NEX)
   B. Number of phase-encoding steps
   C. number of frequency encoding steps
   D. Time of repetition (TR)
   E. Echo train length (ETL)

14 Which of the following would cause a lower signal-to-noise ratio on a T2-weighted image?

   A. Increase the number of averages
   B. Increase the bandwidth
   C. Decrease the echo time (TE)
   D. Decrease the echo train interval

15 A patient has a large, dark-colored tattoo over the area that needs to undergo an MRI examination. Which of the following is a likely safety concern?

   A. Interference with scan
   B. Susceptibility distortion
   C. Heating of the tattoo by radio waves
   D. Heating of the tattoo by gradients

16 The following image of a pelvis has an artifact. What is the most likely cause?

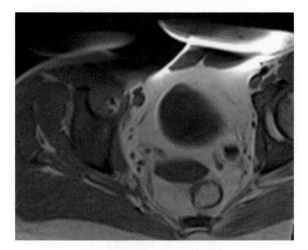

 A. Aliasing of signal from posterior soft tissues
 B. Metal-induced field distortion
 C. Poor fat suppression
 D. Patient movement

17 Why is fluid surrounding the joint hyperintense on this T1-weighted image?

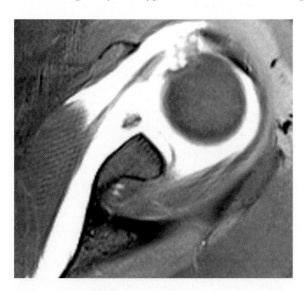

 A. Saline was injected into the joint.
 B. Omnipaque was injected into the joint.
 C. Gadolinium was injected into the joint.
 D. It is an inflow artifact.

18 A 50-year-old male on dialysis presents with findings concerning for osteomyelitis of the foot, and an MRI has been ordered for further characterization. What dose of gadolinium contrast is recommended?

 A. 0.1 mmol/kg
 B. 0.05 mmol/kg
 C. 0.01 mmol/kg
 D. 0 mmol/kg

19 This image of an arm was acquired on a subject with metal in the same arm. Which of the following would exacerbate the artifact?

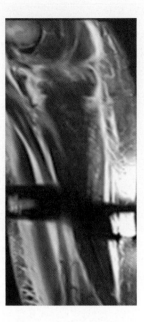

A. Long echo time (TE) gradient-echo sequence
B. Fast/turbo spin echo sequence
C. Short echo time (TE) spin echo sequence
D. Increasing the bandwidth

20 In the image below, the bright signal surrounding the fracture of the distal tibia is best described as which of the following?

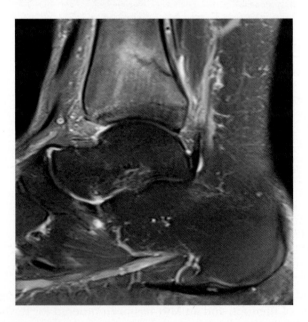

A. Increased T1 signal
B. Increased T2 signal
C. Decreased T1 signal
D. Decreased T2 signal

21 A 35-year-old female undergoes a CT examination with contrast and develops severe bronchospasm. What should you administer?

A. 1 to 3 mL of 1/10,000 dilution of epinephrine IM
B. 1 to 3 mL of 1/10,000 dilution of epinephrine IV
C. 0.3 mL of 1/10,000 dilution of epinephrine IM
D. 0.3 mL of 1/10,000 dilution of epinephrine IV

22 Which of the following is an advantage of performing a biopsy of a soft tissue mass under ultrasound guidance?

A. Allows for the shortest passage of the needle to the target
B. Eliminates the need for conscious sedation
C. Areas of vascularity and viable tissue can be assessed throughout the procedure
D. Allows for use of a smaller gauge biopsy needle

23 Which of the following tumor locations should be biopsied under CT guidance without consideration for ultrasound guidance?

A. Intramedullary
B. Subperiosteal
C. Cortical
D. Soft tissue

24 A 26-year-old male with bacterial endocarditis develops hip pain while in the hospital. A hip aspiration is ordered to evaluate for a septic hip. Which option below represents the most appropriate needle placement for the aspiration?

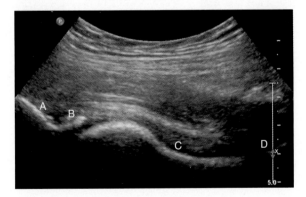

A. A
B. B
C. C
D. D

25 A 20-year-old male endures a wrist injury after a fall. Which of the following studies would offer the best spatial resolution to detect a subtle fracture of the scaphoid cortex?

A. STIR axial images
B. Thin-section CT
C. T1-weighted axial images
D. Bone scan

26 A 75-year-old female with osteoporosis injures her hip after a fall. Which of
the following studies would offer the best contrast resolution to evaluate for a
nondisplaced fracture of the hip?

A. Radiographs
B. CT
C. MRI
D. Ultrasound

27 A 45-year-old male presents with shoulder pain after sustaining an injury
playing tennis. Which of the following studies would offer the best spatial
resolution of the rotator cuff tendons?

A. Bone scan
B. CT
C. MRI
D. Ultrasound

28a A 60-year-old female presents with the dual x-ray absorptiometry study of the
hip presented below. Based on the results of this study, what diagnosis would
this patient receive?

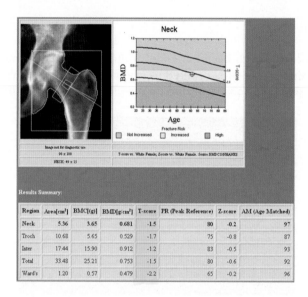

A. Normal
B. Osteomalacia
C. Osteopenia
D. Osteoporosis

28b What is the difference between the T-score and the Z-score?

A. The T-score is the absolute bone mineral density score.
B. The T-score is calculated by comparing the patient to a young-normal
reference population.
C. The Z-score is the absolute bone mineral density score.
D. The Z-score is calculated by comparing the patient to a young-normal
reference population.

29 Which of the following is the most appropriate use of F-18 FDG PET/CT for evaluation of soft tissue tumors?

A. Evaluation of treatment response
B. Biopsy needle placement planning
C. Initial formation of a differential diagnosis
D. Screening of at-risk family members

30 A 45-year-old male presents with clinical concern for vertebral osteomyelitis. The patient has an MRI-incompatible implanted device. Which of the following studies below is suggested for evaluation of vertebral osteomyelitis?

A. Tc-99m MDP
B. Tc-99m HMPAO
C. Ga-67 citrate
D. In-111 WBC

31 A 50-year-old female presents with clinical concern for an infected right knee prosthesis. Which of the following scenarios would be diagnostic for infection?

A. Tc-99m sulfur colloid uptake exceeds In-111 WBC uptake.
B. In-111 WBC uptake exceeds Tc-99m sulfur colloid uptake.
C. Tc-99m sulfur colloid uptake equals In-111 WBC uptake.
D. In-111 WBC has increased uptake without comparison to Tc-99m sulfur colloid.

32 Typically, no grid is used when acquiring extremity radiographs. Which of the following is the best explanation?

A. The use of the grid will block primary x-rays.
B. The use of the grid will degrade image quality.
C. Scatter radiation is not significant in imaging the hand and foot.
D. The use of the grid will decrease patient dose.

33 For anterior to posterior (AP) imaging of the pelvis, which of the following osseous edges will be the sharpest, that is, that has the least blurring (unsharpness)?

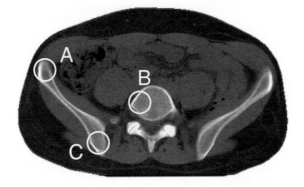

A. A, since it has the longest object to detector distance
B. B, since it is located at the center of the x-ray beam
C. C, since it has the shortest object to detector distance
D. The same, since the focal spot blurring is independent of the location

34   The following images were acquired from the same radiography imaging system. Assuming all other parameters are the same, which of the following will deliver the highest entrance skin exposure to patients?

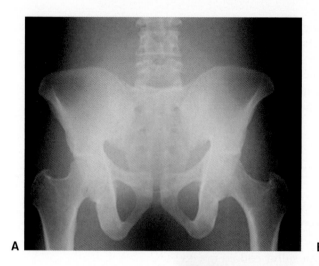
A

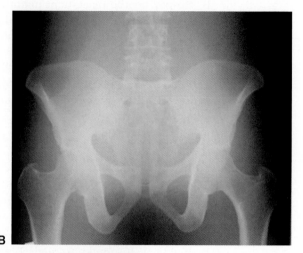
B

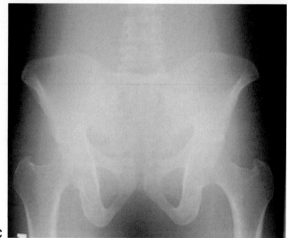
C

A. 60 kV, 130 mAs **B.** 75 kV, 40 mAs **C.** 120 kV, 10 mAs

A. A.
B. B.
C. C.
D. All deliver the same entrance skin exposure.

35   In radiographic imaging, which of the following will result from increasing the x-ray source to detector distance (SID)?

A. Increased focal spot blurring.
B. Decreased focal spot blurring.
C. Increased patient dose.
D. Focal spot blurring is independent of SID.

36 The following image demonstrates metal streak artifact. Changing which of the following acquisition parameters will most efficiently minimize this artifact?

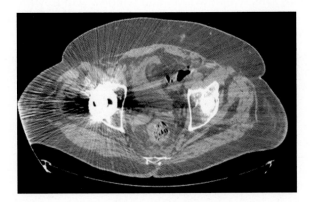

A. Increase kV
B. Decrease kV
C. Increase mAs
D. Decrease mAs

37 The following radiographic image of the chest was obtained with dual-energy subtraction. This technique allows for improved conspicuity of bone abnormalities compared to conventional x-ray images. Dual-energy subtraction is based on the attenuation coefficient changes of bone and soft tissue with x-ray energy. Regarding the attenuation of bone and soft tissues as well as the attenuation difference between the two, which of the following is true when there is an increase of x-ray energy?

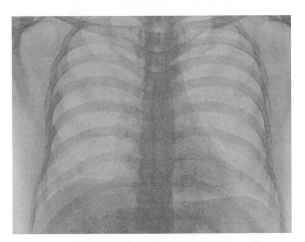

A. Attenuation of bone and tissue both decrease while the attenuation difference decreases.
B. Attenuation of bone and tissue both decrease while the attenuation difference increases.
C. Attenuation of bone and tissue both increase while the attenuation difference decreases.
D. Attenuation of bone and tissue both increase while the attenuation difference increases.

38 The following images are from a patient with a right hip replacement. The images were acquired with the same technical parameters (kV, mAs, pitch) and are shown with same window level and window width. Which of the following is the most likely reason why the first image has less metal hardware artifact than the second?

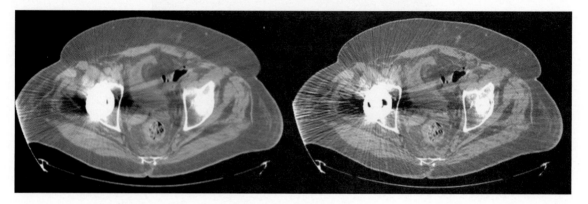

A. Utilization of metal artifact removal software
B. Utilization of different reconstruction kernels
C. Utilization of thicker slices
D. Utilization of thinner slices

39 In the following sagittal image from a cervical spine CT, why is the image quality worse in the lower cervical spine as compared to the upper cervical spine?

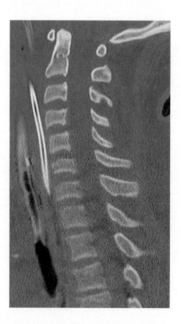

A. Photon starvation at the shoulder area
B. Reconstruction algorithm for sagittal image
C. Larger-size vertebral bodies in the lower cervical spine
D. Patient motion due to breathing during CT acquisition

40 Patient positioning helps improve image quality. Which of the following positions would produce the best radiographic image of the foot?

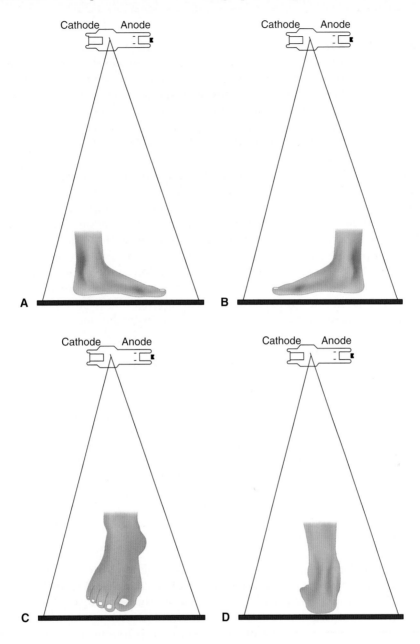

A. A
B. B
C. C
D. D

41 Recently, the Gemstone Spectral Imaging technique was developed, which allows the production of monochromatic spectral images at various voltage levels from dual-energy CT imaging. Why would monochromatic spectral images at high energy be useful in reducing metal artifacts?

A. Monochromatic x-ray photons can substantially reduce beam hardening.
B. Monochromatic x-ray photons can substantially increase beam hardening.
C. Monochromatic x-ray photons can substantially reduce photon starvation.
D. Monochromatic x-ray photons can substantially increase photon starvation.

ANSWERS AND EXPLANATIONS

1   **Answer A.**   Increasing the receiver bandwidth tends to decrease magnetic susceptibility artifact by restricting geometric distortion to a smaller space and overall allowing shorter echo spacing. Increasing field strength, increased voxel size, and increased slice thickness would all tend to increase geometric distortion, and thus worsen susceptibility artifact from metal.

Reference: Bushberg JT, Seibert JA, Leidholdt EM, et al. *The Essential Physics of Medical Imaging*. 3rd ed. Philadelphia, PA: Lippincott Williams & Wilkins; 2012:474–486.

2a   **Answer C.**   The needle is placed on the superomedial humeral head in the rotator interval technique. This position allows the needle tip to be in the region of the rotator interval; therefore, it is superior to the subscapularis tendon and medial and inferior to the supraspinatus tendon. This location allows the needle tip to avoid piercing either tendon. If the needle tip was placed at position D, it may pierce the supraspinatus tendon. The needle is not placed on the glenoid side of the joint. In addition to the rotator cuff interval approach, the needle may be placed into the glenohumeral articulation via an anterior or posterior approach. The junction of the middle and inferior two-thirds of the glenohumeral joint is targeted in this technique.

References: Crim J, Morrison WB. *Specialty Imaging: Arthrography: Principles and Practice in Radiology*. Salt Lake City, UT: Amirsys; 2009:24–27.
Peterson JJ, Fenton DS, Czervinoke LF. *Image-Guided Musculoskeletal Intervention*. Philadelphia, PA: Saunders; 2008:27–31.

2b   **Answer A.**   The most appropriate choice of contrast mixture is iodinated contrast 1:1 with saline and/or anesthetic. If considerably less iodinated contrast is used, the mixture may not be well visualized either on the arthrogram or on the following CT examination, rendering the study essentially an anesthetic/saline injection without the benefit of iodinated contrast.

References: Crim J, Morrison WB. *Specialty Imaging: Arthrography: Principles and Practice in Radiology*. Salt Lake City, UT: Amirsys; 2009:2–3.
Peterson JJ, Fenton DS, Czervinoke LF. *Image-Guided Musculoskeletal Intervention*. Philadelphia, PA: Saunders; 2008:27.

2c   **Answer D.**   Reasons for performing a CT arthrogram instead of an MRI arthrogram include contraindications to MRI, such as metal near the joint in question. Postoperative rotator cuff evaluation can be performed with either MRI or CT. Anticoagulation and infection at the joint are contraindications for arthrography in general regardless of whether it is followed by CT or MRI. Lack of joint mobility does not necessarily negate the ability to perform a shoulder MRI, however, certain sequences such as the ABER (abduction, external rotation) view may not be possible. In this case, a posterior superior labral tear is noted.

Reference: Weissman BN. *Imaging of Arthritis and Metabolic Bone Disease*. Philadelphia, PA: Saunders; 2009:60–66.

3   **Answer D.**   The farther a coil is from the area of interest, the lower the signal, and thus the lower the overall signal-to-noise ratio since noise is constant. Receiver bandwidth and spatial resolution parameters are independent of the signal-to-noise ratio.

Reference: Bushberg JT, Seibert JA, Leidholdt EM, et al. *The Essential Physics of Medical Imaging*. 3rd ed. Philadelphia, PA: Lippincott Williams & Wilkins; 2012:460–464.

4   Answer A.   Compartment syndrome would be the primary clinical concern following infiltration of a large volume of IV contrast. NSF is a chronic adverse reaction to gadolinium. Renal dysfunction can occur following IV administration of iodinated contrast, typically occurring several days following the contrast dose.

Reference: American College of Radiology (ACR). *ACR Manual on Contrast Media*. Version 9. Reston, VA: American College of Radiology; 2013:17–20.

5   Answer B.   30% to 40% of the bone mineralization must be lost to be visualized by radiographs. Radiographs are insensitive in detecting early bone loss.

Reference: Weissman BN. *Imaging of Arthritis and Metabolic Bone Disease*. Philadelphia, PA: Saunders; 2009:608.

6a   Answer D.   Three approaches have been described for entering the hip joint: direct vertical, oblique (lateral to medial) vertical, and lateral which targets the lateral margin of the femoral head. The most commonly performed approaches are the direct vertical and oblique vertical. The advantage of the direct vertical is that the needle remains parallel to the fluoroscopic beam, thus allowing for simple and straightforward entry into the joint. The preferred location for needle placement in the direct vertical approach is on the superior lateral head–neck junction of the femur. This is denoted by D on the image. B is another possible location, but this location is close to the vessels and femoral nerve and may lead to an iliopsoas injection. The needle is not placed into the femoroacetabular joint or on the acetabular side of the joint; therefore, A and C are incorrect.

References: Crim J, Morrison WB. *Specialty Imaging: Arthrography: Principles and Practice in Radiology*. Salt Lake City, UT: Amirsys; 2009:130–133.
Peterson JJ, Fenton DS, Czervinoke LF. *Image-Guided Musculoskeletal Intervention*. Philadelphia, PA: Saunders; 2008:95–98.

6b   Answer B.   The correct mixture is 0.1 to 0.2 mL gadolinium per 20 mL of iodinated contrast, saline, and/or anesthetic. Gadolinium is therefore diluted to a 1/100–1/200 concentration. If the gadolinium is not dilute enough it appears as a low signal fluid collection obscuring the relevant findings. If the gadolinium is too dilute, the appearance is more comparable to a saline arthrogram.

References: Crim J, Morrison WB. *Specialty Imaging: Arthrography: Principles and Practice in Radiology*. Salt Lake City, UT: Amirsys; 2009:2–3.
Peterson JJ, Fenton DS, Czervinoke LF. *Image-Guided Musculoskeletal Intervention*. Philadelphia, PA: Saunders; 2008:1–5.

6c   Answer B.   MRI arthrography is advantageous for evaluation of labral tears, cartilage defects, osteochondral bodies, and ligamentum teres injuries and monitoring hip dysplasias. CT arthrography may be beneficial in large or obese patients, in postoperative evaluation of labral tears to avoid the metallic artifact seen in labral repair on MRI, and in patients who cannot undergo MRI evaluation. In this case, an anterior superior labral tear is seen with an associated paralabral cyst.

Reference: Weissman BN. *Imaging of Arthritis and Metabolic Bone Disease*. Philadelphia, PA: Saunders; 2009:62–68.

7   Answer B.   The artifact shown is aliasing in the phase-encoding direction resulting in the subject's left leg being superimposed on the anatomy of the right leg. By doubling the image oversampling in the phase-encoded direction, this artifact will be eliminated.

Reference: Bushberg JT, Seibert JA, Leidholdt EM, et al. *The Essential Physics of Medical Imaging*. 3rd ed. Philadelphia, PA: Lippincott Williams & Wilkins; 2012:474–486.

8   **Answer C.**   Fluid is bright on a T2-weighted image. Liquids have long T2 relaxation times, whereas solids generally have short T2 relaxation. Tissues with a long T2 relaxation time will be bright on T2-weighted images, whereas tissues with a short T1 relaxation time will be bright on T1-weighted imaging.

Reference: Bushberg JT, Seibert JA, Leidholdt EM, et al. *The Essential Physics of Medical Imaging*. 3rd ed. Philadelphia, PA: Lippincott Williams & Wilkins; 2012:425–427.

9   **Answer B.**   Imaging at high resolution requires thin slices; however, when you use thin slices in a 2D acquisition, the signal-to-noise tends to decrease too much for the images to be useful. This decrease can be overcome using 3D, which achieves thin slices but regains SNR through averaging.

Reference: Bushberg JT, Seibert JA, Leidholdt EM, et al. *The Essential Physics of Medical Imaging*. 3rd ed. Philadelphia, PA: Lippincott Williams & Wilkins; 2012:459–460.

10   **Answer C.**   The radial imaging techniques such as BLADE (MRI acronym, Siemens) and PROPELLOR (MRI acronym, GE) sample the center of k-space more frequently than standard rectilinear techniques. As a result, they can tolerate more movement of patients during the image acquisition without significantly degrading the image quality.

Reference: Bushberg JT, Seibert JA, Leidholdt EM, et al. *The Essential Physics of Medical Imaging*. 3rd ed. Philadelphia, PA: Lippincott Williams & Wilkins; 2012:456–457.

11   **Answer A.**   Gibbs phenomenon, also known as ringing artifact, has the appearance of multiple, regularly spaced bands that are parallel to one another. They typically present as alternating bright and dark signal bands that slowly fade as the distance from the source of the artifact increases. They often occur at sharp boundaries, which have high contrast transitions in the image. This artifact is caused by insufficient sampling of high frequencies, which may occur at sharp discontinuities in signal.

Reference: Bushberg JT, Seibert JA, Leidholdt EM, et al. *The Essential Physics of Medical Imaging*. 3rd ed. Philadelphia, PA: Lippincott Williams & Wilkins; 2012:483–484.

12   **Answer A.**   A circulating gadolinium contrast agent will accumulate in the sarcoma and cause a decrease in the T1 relaxation time. This decrease will result in the sarcoma appearing bright on the T1-weighted image. Tissues with a short T1 relaxation time will be bright on T1-weighted imaging, whereas tissues with a long T2 relaxation time will be bright on T2-weighted images.

Reference: Bushberg JT, Seibert JA, Leidholdt EM, et al. *The Essential Physics of Medical Imaging*. 3rd ed. Philadelphia, PA: Lippincott Williams & Wilkins; 2012:423–424.

13   **Answer C.**   Total scan time is directly proportional to time of repetition (TR), number of excitations (NEX), and number of phase-encoding steps. Total scan time is inversely proportional to the echo train length (ETL). The number of frequency-encoding steps does not alter acquisition time.

Reference: Bushberg JT, Seibert JA, Leidholdt EM, et al. *The Essential Physics of Medical Imaging*. 3rd ed. Philadelphia, PA: Lippincott Williams & Wilkins; 2012:450.

14   **Answer B.**   The signal-to-noise ratio is proportional to the inverse square root of the frequency-encoded bandwidth. Thus, increasing the bandwidth increases the amount of noise collected and will decrease the signal-to-noise ratio.

Reference: Bushberg JT, Seibert JA, Leidholdt EM, et al. *The Essential Physics of Medical Imaging*. 3rd ed. Philadelphia, PA: Lippincott Williams & Wilkins; 2012:440–441.

15   **Answer C.**   The safety concern would be heating of the tattoo by absorption of radiofrequency waves because the tattoo may contain small fragments of metal.

This contamination is more common in older tattoos, but is uncommon in the newer inks used in tattooing over the last 20 years.

Reference: Bushberg JT, Seibert JA, Leidholdt EM, et al. *The Essential Physics of Medical Imaging.* 3rd ed. Philadelphia, PA: Lippincott Williams & Wilkins; 2012:495–499.

16 **Answer B.** The artifact in the image results from the metal on the patient's lower abdomen, such as a pants' zipper.

Reference: Bushberg JT, Seibert JA, Leidholdt EM, et al. *The Essential Physics of Medical Imaging.* 3rd ed. Philadelphia, PA: Lippincott Williams & Wilkins; 2012:474–486.

17 **Answer C.** T1 relaxation time is long in water molecules, and thus fluid is hypointense on T1. This T1-weighted image represents an arthrogram where gadolinium contrast has been injected into the joint. The fluid surrounding the joint is hyperintense on this T1-weighted image, because gadolinium causes T1 shortening. Saline and omnipaque would appear as increased signal on a T2-weighted image, but not on a T1-weighted image.

Reference: Bushberg JT, Seibert JA, Leidholdt EM, et al. *The Essential Physics of Medical Imaging.* 3rd ed. Philadelphia, PA: Lippincott Williams & Wilkins; 2012:423–426.

18 **Answer D.** Though there are some MRI-compatible contrast agents that can be considered in dialysis patients, gadolinium injection for MRI contrast examinations is typically to be avoided in patients on dialysis for fear of nephrogenic systemic fibrosis (NSF). This is particularly true in the case of osteomyelitis in which the diagnosis may be reached without the use of contrast. Additional patients who are considered at risk for NSF include those with severe or end-stage chronic kidney disease without dialysis, eGFR 30 to 40 mL/min/1.73 m² without dialysis, and acute kidney injury superimposed on chronic kidney disease.

Reference: American College of Radiology (ACR). *ACR Manual on Contrast Media.* Version 9. Reston, VA: American College of Radiology; 2013:81–90.

19 **Answer A.** The presence of the metal induces substantial inhomogeneity in the magnetic field. Gradient-echo images are particularly sensitive to magnetic field inhomogeneities because they do not have a 180-degree pulse to refocus the magnetization. This effect is exacerbated with longer echo times.

Reference: Bushberg JT, Seibert JA, Leidholdt EM, et al. *The Essential Physics of Medical Imaging.* 3rd ed. Philadelphia, PA: Lippincott Williams & Wilkins; 2012:431–437.

20 **Answer B.** The image is T2 weighted with fat saturation. The bright signal surrounding the fracture results from increased bone edema and thus increased T2 signal.

Reference: Bushberg JT, Seibert JA, Leidholdt EM, et al. *The Essential Physics of Medical Imaging.* 3rd ed. Philadelphia, PA: Lippincott Williams & Wilkins; 2012:425–427.

21 **Answer B.** Reactions to iodinated contrast for which epinephrine treatment should be considered include severe hives, diffuse erythema with hypotension, moderate or severe bronchospasm, all forms of laryngeal edema, persistent hypotension, and those who are unresponsive and pulseless. The correct dose of epinephrine is either 1 to 3 mL of 1/10,000 dilution IV or 0.3 mL of 1/1,000 dilution IM.

Reference: American College of Radiology (ACR). *ACR Manual on Contrast Media.* Version 9. Reston, VA: American College of Radiology; 2013:103–109.

22 **Answer C.** Many factors are similar when performing a biopsy under ultrasound guidance as compared to another modality, such as CT guidance. The need for conscious sedation, the type of needle used, and the path to the target may all be similar whether using ultrasound or CT guidance. An advantage of ultrasound is the ability to use color Doppler throughout a procedure to detect vessels as well as areas of a mass that are more vascular. IV contrast may be given prior to or during a CT-guided procedure to identify vessels and enhancing areas of tumor, but the contrast will dissipate and is contraindicated in some patients. The vascular area of the tumor represents viable tissue and should be targeted, as opposed to the areas without vascularization that may represent necrosis. Other advantages of US include the lack of radiation, potential improved patient satisfaction with positioning, real-time visualization of the needle, and potential increased speed of the biopsy. As with any biopsy in musculoskeletal radiology, discussion with the orthopedic surgeon to determine the approach prior to biopsy is recommended to avoid inappropriate tissue contamination and more aggressive surgery. Needles for ultrasound-guided sampling may include 22 gauge for fine needle aspiration or 14 to 18 gauge for core biopsy.

Reference: Bianchi S, Martinoli C. *Ultrasound of the Musculoskeletal System*. Berlin, Germany: Springer; 2007:896–897.

23 Answer A. Many masses can be biopsied under ultrasound guidance. Soft tissue masses are often easily targeted with ultrasound guidance. Cortical or subperiosteal lesions are potentially visible with ultrasound guidance as well, particularly if the cortex is broken. Intramedullary lesions are best approached utilizing CT guidance.

Reference: Bianchi S, Martinoli C. *Ultrasound of the Musculoskeletal System*. Berlin, Germany: Springer; 2007:896–897.

24 Answer C. The image presented is a long-axis, or sagittal, image of the left hip using a curvilinear transducer. A marks the acetabulum, B marks the labrum, and D marks the proximal femur inferior to the joint capsule. The needle should not be placed onto the acetabular side of the joint, within the labrum, or inferior to the joint capsule on the proximal femur. C marks the anterior recess of the femoral head neck junction and represents the most appropriate position to place the needle for a hip aspiration or injection under ultrasound guidance.

Reference: Bianchi S, Martinoli C. *Ultrasound of the Musculoskeletal System*. Berlin, Germany: Springer; 2007:908–909.

25 Answer B. The cortical surfaces of the scaphoid traverse many planes and multiple angles, making detection of a subtle fracture of the scaphoid difficult with radiographs. Spatial resolution is the ability to differentiate between two high-contrast objects. Currently, CT offers the best spatial resolution for detection of subtle fractures of the cortex.

Reference: Weissman BN. *Imaging of Arthritis and Metabolic Bone Disease*. Philadelphia, PA: Saunders; 2009:3–6.

26 Answer C. MRI offers the best contrast resolution for detection of nondisplaced hip fractures. Contrast resolution is the ability to detect differences in intensities in adjacent regions on an image. In the hip, this would allow the detection of a nondisplaced fracture line, bone marrow edema, and hemorrhage.

Reference: Weissman BN. *Imaging of Arthritis and Metabolic Bone Disease*. Philadelphia, PA: Saunders; 2009:3–6.

27 Answer D. With the aid of high-resolution transducers, ultrasound currently offers the best spatial resolution for evaluation of superficial structures such as many ligaments and tendons. In the shoulder, the rotator cuff is well visualized in most patients with the use of ultrasound utilizing transducers ranging from 7.5 to 20 MHz. The resolving power of current ultrasound units is <0.1 mm, which is better than either CT or MRI.

Reference: Weissman BN. *Imaging of Arthritis and Metabolic Bone Disease*. Philadelphia, PA: Saunders; 2009:90.

28a **Answer C.** The T-score is most commonly used for diagnosis. According to the World Health Organization Criteria, a normal bone mineral density has a T-score ≥-1.0, osteopenia is between -1.0 and -2.5, and osteoporosis is ≤-2.5. In this case, the T-score is in the range of osteopenia. When diagnosing osteoporosis, the lower of the T-scores between the PA spine (not shown in this case) and the hip is used. When evaluating the hip for fracture risk, the lower of the T-scores of the hip should be used.

Reference: Weissman BN. *Imaging of Arthritis and Metabolic Bone Disease*. Philadelphia, PA: Saunders; 2009:81–88.

28b **Answer B.** Absolute bone mineral density (BMD) measurements are not used for the diagnosis of osteoporosis. Instead, T-score values are used for diagnosis. The T-score is a standardized score calculated by subtracting the BMD of a young-normal reference population from the patient's measured BMD and dividing by the standard deviation of a young-normal reference population. A Z-score is calculated similar to a T-score, except the patient is compared against an age-matched reference population instead of a young-normal reference population.

Reference: Weissman BN. *Imaging of Arthritis and Metabolic Bone Disease*. Philadelphia, PA: Saunders; 2009:81–88.

29 **Answer A.** F-18 FDG PET/CT imaging has several potential uses in malignant soft tissue tumors, including primary staging, metastatic evaluation, and evaluation of tumor response to treatment. It does not currently have a role in biopsy needle placement planning or as a screening exam. Although it has shown promise in distinguishing high-grade sarcomas, it is not currently routine clinical practice to use FDG-PET in the initial formation of a differential diagnosis.

References: Beaman FD, Jelinek JS, Priebat DA. Current imaging and therapy of malignant soft tissue tumors and tumor-like lesions. *Semin Musculoskelet Radiol*. 2013;17:168–176.
Weissman BN. *Imaging of Arthritis and Metabolic Bone Disease*. Philadelphia, PA: Saunders; 2009:30–32.

30 **Answer C.** Ga-67 citrate is the preferred study for evaluation of discitis osteomyelitis. SPECT imaging can be used with Ga-67 citrate to increase its sensitivity. The other studies may be used but are not preferred over Ga-67 citrate.

References: Love C, Patel M, Lonner BS, et al. Diagnosing spinal osteomyelitis: a comparison of bone and Ga-67 scintigraphy and magnetic resonance imaging. *Clin Nucl Med*. 2000;25(12):963–977.
Weissman BN. *Imaging of Arthritis and Metabolic Bone Disease*. Philadelphia, PA: Saunders; 2009:20–21.

31 **Answer B.** Diagnosing infection in prosthesis patients can be performed with a Tc-99m sulfur colloid and In-111 WBC combined study. In this study, the Tc-99m sulfur colloid uptake is subtracted, either visually or with the aid of a computer, from the In-111 WBC uptake. If the In-111 WBC uptake exceeds the Tc-99m sulfur colloid uptake, the study is considered positive for infection. An In-111 WBC scan is not performed alone because false-positive results may occur due to physiologic uptake from the marrow. By performing the combined study, this physiologic uptake is corrected as it will be present on both studies and will therefore be subtracted out.

Reference: Weissman BN. *Imaging of Arthritis and Metabolic Bone Disease*. Philadelphia, PA: Saunders; 2009:22–23.

32   **Answer C.**   Scatter radiation depends on the size of the imaging area and the patient's size. For small body regions, less radiation is generated.

Reference: Bushberg JT, Seibert JA, Leidholdt EM, et al. *The Essential Physics of Medical Imaging*. 3rd ed. Philadelphia, PA: Lippincott Williams & Wilkins; 2012:231–235.

33   **Answer C.**   Focal spot blurring depends on geometric structure. It is directly proportional to the object to detector distance and inversely proportional to the x-ray source to object distance. C has the shortest object to detector distance and the longest source to object distance, compared to A and B.

Reference: Bushberg JT, Seibert JA, Leidholdt EM, et al. *The Essential Physics of Medical Imaging*. 3rd ed. Philadelphia, PA: Lippincott Williams & Wilkins; 2012:207–209.

34   **Answer A.**   X-ray intensity (measured by exposure) is proportional to the square of kV and proportional to mAs. Increasing kV while decreasing mAs potentially helps reduce radiation dose.

Reference: Bushberg JT, Seibert JA, Leidholdt EM, et al. *The Essential Physics of Medical Imaging*. 3rd ed. Philadelphia, PA: Lippincott Williams & Wilkins; 2012:202–206.

35   **Answer B.**   Focal spot blurring depends on geometric structure. It is directly proportional to object to detector distance and inversely proportional to x-ray source to object distance. Increasing SID will increase x-ray to object distance, while object to detector distance remains the same.

Reference: Bushberg JT, Seibert JA, Leidholdt EM, et al. *The Essential Physics of Medical Imaging*. 3rd ed. Philadelphia, PA: Lippincott Williams & Wilkins; 2012:207–209.

36   **Answer A.**   The presence of metal objects in the scan field can lead to severe streak artifact. This artifact is due to incomplete attenuation profiles where the density of the metal is beyond the normal range. Increasing kV can help penetrate the object, thereby decreasing the streak artifact.

Reference: Bushberg JT, Seibert JA, Leidholdt EM, et al. *The Essential Physics of Medical Imaging*. 3rd ed. Philadelphia, PA: Lippincott Williams & Wilkins; 2012:367–370.

37   **Answer A.**   With the increase of x-ray energy, attenuation always decreases, and the attenuation difference between different materials will also decrease.

Reference: Bushberg JT, Seibert JA, Leidholdt EM, et al. *The Essential Physics of Medical Imaging*. 3rd ed. Philadelphia, PA: Lippincott Williams & Wilkins; 2012:228–230.

38   **Answer C.**   Increasing reconstruction slice thickness helps reduce metal artifact. In general, the use of metal artifact removal software changes the artifact pattern. In this question, the images show the same metal artifact pattern; therefore, metal artifact removal software was not used. The use of a smooth reconstruction kernel may also help reduce artifacts but will not change the partial volume effect. Here, the first image shows greater partial volume effect compared to the second image.

Reference: Bushberg JT, Seibert JA, Leidholdt EM, et al. *The Essential Physics of Medical Imaging*. 3rd ed. Philadelphia, PA: Lippincott Williams & Wilkins; 2012:367–370.

39 Answer A.   Insufficient x-ray photons arrive at the detector at the lower cervical levels because of the patient's large shoulders, which is known as photon starvation.

Reference: Bushberg JT, Seibert JA, Leidholdt EM, et al. *The Essential Physics of Medical Imaging.* 3rd ed. Philadelphia, PA: Lippincott Williams & Wilkins; 2012:367–370.

40 Answer A.   The heel effect: X-ray intensity on the cathode side of the x-ray field is higher than that on the anode side. The difference in radiation intensity across the useful beam of an x-ray field can vary by as much as 45%. The heel effect is important when imaging anatomic structures that differ greatly in thickness or mass density. In general, positioning the cathode side over the thicker part of the anatomy provides more uniform exposure to the detector. Therefore, the calcaneus should be on the cathode side.

Reference: Bushberg JT, Seibert JA, Leidholdt EM, et al. *The Essential Physics of Medical Imaging.* 3rd ed. Philadelphia, PA: Lippincott Williams & Wilkins; 2012:184–185.

41 Answer A.   In general, the beam is composed of individual photons with a range of energies. As the beam passes through an object, it becomes "harder," meaning the energy increases, because the lower-energy photons are absorbed more rapidly, leaving behind only the high-energy photons. For a monochromatic beam, no energy change is involved.

Reference: Bushberg JT, Seibert JA, Leidholdt EM, et al. *The Essential Physics of Medical Imaging.* 3rd ed. Philadelphia, PA: Lippincott Williams & Wilkins; 2012:367–370.

2   Normal/Normal Variants

QUESTIONS

1   What is the most common location for the imaged finding?

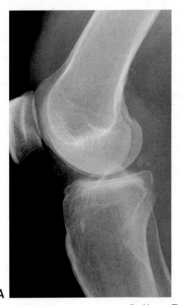 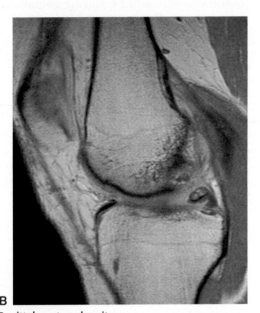

A. X-ray **B.** Sagittal proton density

A. Posterior horn of the lateral meniscus
B. Anterior horn of the lateral meniscus
C. Posterior horn of the medial meniscus
D. Anterior horn of the medial meniscus

2 A 62-year-old female presents with a radial head fracture. What is noted by the arrow on the images below?

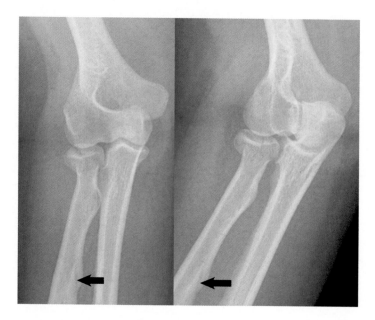

    A. Nondisplaced fracture
    B. Nutrient channel
    C. Origin of flexor digitorum profundus muscle
    D. Groove for the median nerve

3 A 62-year-old female presents with trauma of her right arm. What is the most likely cause for the alignment of the radius and ulna?

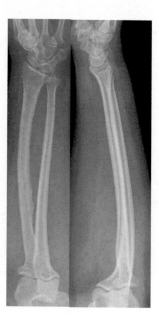

    A. Physiologic bowing
    B. Dislocation of the radial head
    C. Dislocation of the distal ulna
    D. Greenstick fracture of the radius and ulna

4   Regarding the lucency in the humeral head, what is the next most appropriate imaging study?

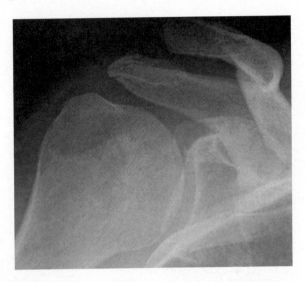

- A. Additional radiographs
- B. CT
- C. MRI
- D. Nuclear medicine bone scan

5   A 14-year-old male presents with pain in his knee after a sports-related injury. What is noted by the arrows on the image below?

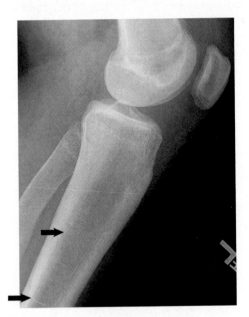

- A. Stress fracture
- B. Lead lines
- C. Transverse growth lines
- D. Metaphyseal lines

6 An 11-year-old male presents with knee pain. A periosteal desmoid is incidentally noted. Which option below correctly describes the classic location for this finding?

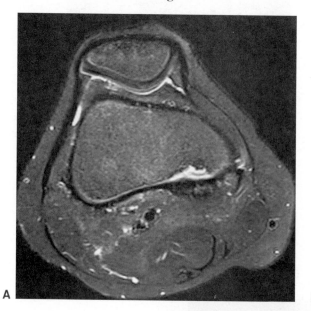

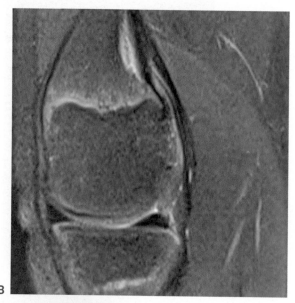

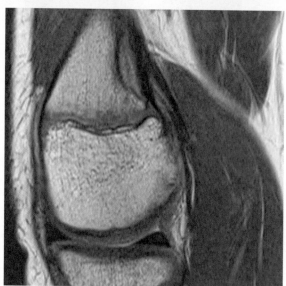

A. Axial T2 fat saturation **B.** Sagittal T2 fat saturation **C.** Sagittal proton density

A. Insertion of the semitendinosus tendon
B. Origin of the popliteus tendon
C. Insertion of the semimembranosus tendon
D. Origin of the medial head of the gastrocnemius tendon

7a What structure is noted by the arrows on the images below?

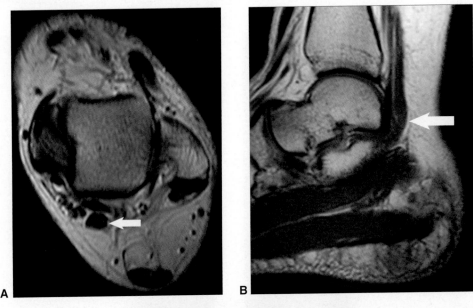

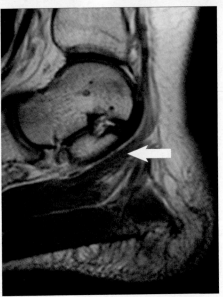

A. Axial proton density **B.** Sagittal T1 weighted **C.** Sagittal T1 weighted

   A. Peroneus quartus muscle
   B. Accessory soleus muscle
   C. Accessory flexor digitorum longus muscle
   D. Plantaris muscle

7b What is the most common accessory muscle of the ankle?

   A. Peroneus quartus
   B. Accessory soleus
   C. Accessory flexor digitorum longus
   D. Peroneocalcaneus internus

8 A 15-year-old male pitcher presents with pain in the pitching elbow. What is the most likely cause of the finding noted?

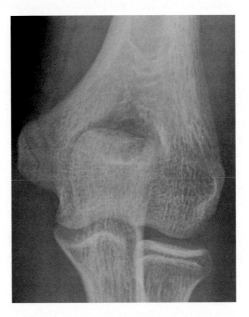

A. Medial epicondylitis at the common flexor tendon origin
B. Avulsion of the medial epicondyle at the ulnar collateral ligament attachment
C. Avulsion of the sublime tubercle at the ulnar collateral ligament attachment
D. Incompletely fused medial epicondyle

ANSWERS AND EXPLANATIONS

1 **Answer C.** Along with the fabella and cyamella, the meniscal ossicle is one of the three most common sesamoid bones and ossicles of the knee. It is most commonly seen in the posterior horn of the medial meniscus. It usually presents in young men. It is seen in <1% of knee examinations. On radiographs, it presents as a triangular opacity at the periphery of the meniscus. MR, CT, and ultrasound will demonstrate an intrameniscal location.

Reference: Yochum T, Rowe L. *Essentials of Skeletal Radiology.* 3rd ed. Philadelphia, PA: Lippincott Williams & Wilkins; 2005:332.

2 **Answer B.** The lucency in the cortex of the radius is the classic location for the nutrient channel. It is important to know this normal structure to avoid describing a fracture for this finding.

Reference: Keats TE, Anderson MW. *Atlas of Normal Roentgen Variants That May Simulate Disease.* 7th ed. St. Louis, MO: Mosby; 2001:522.

3 **Answer A.** The alignment of the radius and ulna is associated with physiologic bowing. This finding is often seen in the setting of negative ulnar variance, which this patient has but is somewhat difficult to detect on the provided images.

Reference: Keats TE, Anderson MW. *Atlas of Normal Roentgen Variants That May Simulate Disease.* 7th ed. St. Louis, MO: Mosby; 2001:523.

4 **Answer A.** The lucency in the humeral head has a cyst-like appearance; however, this is the classic location for the pseudolesion of the humeral head, which is typically noted on internal rotation views of the shoulder. Additional radiographic views, such as an external rotation view, will not demonstrate a similar finding, indicating this finding is not a true lesion.

Reference: Keats TE, Anderson MW. *Atlas of Normal Roentgen Variants That May Simulate Disease.* 7th ed. St. Louis, MO: Mosby; 2001:480.

5 **Answer C.** The lines are thin, sclerotic bands in the proximal metaphysis of the tibia. They are transverse growth lines and typically reflect prior osteoblastic activity during the recovery phase after an illness. Metaphyseal lines, on the other hand, are dense lines at the zone of provisional calcification immediately adjacent to the physis and do not extend into the proximal metaphysis. Stress fractures are seen as a lucency in the cortex of the bone, while lead lines are dense metaphyseal lines, often seen in the knee and wrist.

Reference: Siegel MJ, Coley BD. *The Core Curriculum: Pediatric Imaging.* Philadelphia, PA: Lippincott Williams & Wilkins; 2006:409–410.

6 **Answer D.** Periosteal desmoid has many other names, including avulsive cortical irregularity, distal metaphyseal femoral defect, cortical desmoid, and medial supracondylar defect of the femur. The finding is characteristically seen in the posteromedial cortex of the distal end of the femur, adjacent to the medial femoral condyle. It is located at the insertion of the adductor magnus aponeurosis or the origin of the medial head of the gastrocnemius tendon. It is typically seen in patients ages 15 to 20 years and may be a reaction to trauma. On radiographs, it demonstrates a saucer-like lucent defect. It is typically hypointense on T1-weighted MR images and hyperintense on T2-weighted MR images. It is a benign finding, and no further imaging is needed.

References: Greenspan A, Gernot J, Wolfgang R. *Differential Diagnosis in Orthopaedic Oncology*. 2nd ed. Philadelphia, PA: Lippincott Williams & Wilkins; 2007:267–270.
Resnick D, Kang HS, Pretterklieber ML. *Internal Derangements of Joints*. 2nd ed. Philadelphia, PA: Saunders; 2007:469–470.

7a **Answer C.** The arrow points to the accessory flexor digitorum longus. The three normal tendons of the medial ankle are visualized separate from this structure, indicating this is an accessory muscle. There are three accessory muscles, which can be seen in the medial ankle: the accessory flexor digitorum longus, accessory soleus, and peroneocalcaneus internus. Of these, only the accessory soleus is located superficial to the flexor retinaculum outside of the tarsal tunnel. The most common accessory muscle seen in the lateral ankle is the peroneus quartus.

Reference: Resnick D, Kang HS, Pretterklieber ML. *Internal Derangements of Joints*. 2nd ed. Philadelphia, PA: Saunders; 2007:523–524.

7b **Answer A.** The most common accessory muscle is the peroneus quartus, occurring in up to 10% to 22% of the population. The accessory flexor digitorum longus occurs in 2% to 8% of the population. The accessory soleus occurs in 1% to 6% of the population, while the peroneocalcaneus internus occurs in 1% of the population.

Reference: Resnick D, Kang HS, Pretterklieber ML. *Internal Derangements of Joints*. 2nd ed. Philadelphia, PA: Saunders; 2007:523–524.

8 **Answer B.** The order of ossification of the elbow begins with the capitellum at ~1 to 2 years of age, radius at 3 years, medial epicondyle at 4 years, trochlea at 8 years, and lateral epicondyle at 10 years. This patient is 15 years old; therefore, the elbow should be ossified. There is a lucency noted in the medial epicondyle, which, given the history of a throwing athlete, is most consistent with an avulsion of the medial epicondyle at the ulnar collateral ligament attachment. In younger patients, before there is complete ossification of the elbow, a similar injury can be caused by avulsion from excessive pull of the common flexor tendon. The ulnar attachment of the ulnar collateral ligament is the sublime tubercle; however, no radiographic abnormality is noted in this location. Medial epicondylitis is related to tendinosis of the common flexor tendon and would not cause the finding noted in this patient.

References: Resnick D, Kang HS, Pretterklieber ML. *Internal Derangements of Joints*. 2nd ed. Philadelphia, PA: Saunders; 2007:1189–1193.
Siegel MJ, Coley BD. *The Core Curriculum: Pediatric Imaging*. Philadelphia, PA: Lippincott Williams & Wilkins; 2006:510–513.

Congenital and Developmental Spine/Extremity Anomalies and Dysplasias

QUESTIONS

1 A 4-year-old male presented to the emergency room with pain. These radiographs were obtained and preliminarily reported as fracture. What is the most likely diagnosis?

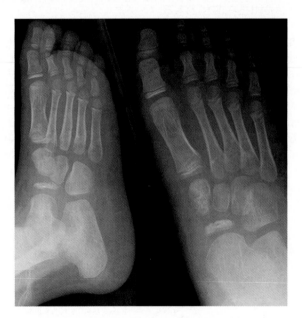

A. Freiberg infraction
B. Insufficiency fracture
C. Köhler disease
D. Lisfranc injury

2 What is the most common carpal coalition?

A. Scapholunate
B. Scaphotrapeziotrapezoidal
C. Lunotriquetral
D. Capitate–hamate

3   The radiograph demonstrates what wrist abnormality?

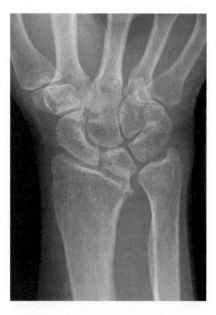

   A. Scapholunate advanced collapse (SLAC wrist)
   B. Kienböck disease
   C. Perilunate dislocation
   D. Madelung deformity

4   Plexiform neurofibromas are most commonly seen in which of the following syndromes?

   A. Neurofibromatosis type 1
   B. Neurofibromatosis type 2
   C. Sturge-Weber
   D. Tuberous sclerosis

5a   A 30-year-old male presents with the following radiograph. The abnormality most commonly results in which one of the following clinical symptoms?

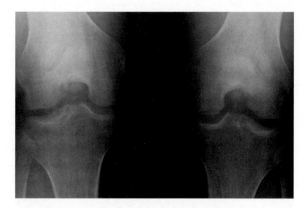

   A. Anterior knee pain
   B. Lateral knee pain
   C. Inability to fully extend the knee
   D. Inability to fully flex the knee

5b   What is the most common MRI finding in this anomaly?

   A. Quadriceps tendinosis
   B. Patellar tendinosis
   C. Hyperintense T2 signal within the bipartite fragment
   D. Nonenhancement of the bipartite fragment suggesting devitalized bone

6   Which one of the following clinical manifestations is associated with the syndrome depicted by the CT and radiograph below?

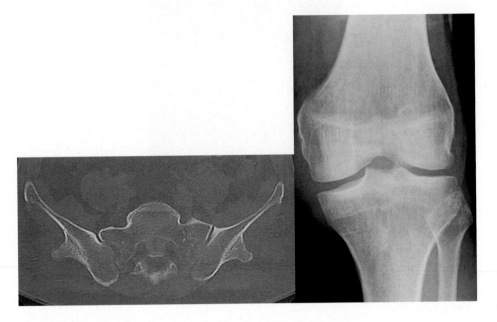

   A. Ataxia
   B. Nail changes
   C. Hypertension
   D. Arrhythmias

7   Which of the following would be included in the differential diagnosis for the findings noted in the image below?

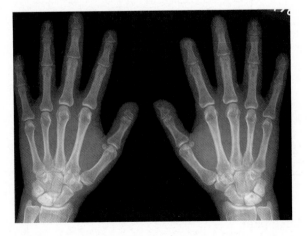

   A. Congenital insensitivity to pain
   B. Hypoparathyroidism
   C. Hyperthyroidism
   D. Osteoarthrosis

8 Bridging ossification between osseous structures in fibrodysplasia ossificans progressiva typically occurs where initially?

A. Pelvis
B. Sternocleidomastoid
C. Shoulder girdle
D. Upper arms

9 A patient presents with enlargement of the second and third digits of the right hand. On radiographs of the right hand, there is osseous overgrowth of the second and third digit, long and broad phalanges, splayed distal tufts, bowing deformity, and enlargement of the soft tissues. What is the most likely diagnosis?

A. Dermatomyositis
B. Scleroderma
C. Macrodystrophia lipomatosa
D. Leprosy

10 Which of the findings below is more commonly seen in primary hypertrophic osteoarthropathy as compared to secondary hypertrophic osteoarthropathy?

A. Phalangeal tuft hypertrophy
B. Phalangeal tuft acroosteolysis
C. Phalangeal tuft sparring
D. Phalangeal tuft sclerosis

11 A 21-year-old male presents with back pain. Which of the following is correctly associated with the diagnosis depicted by the image below?

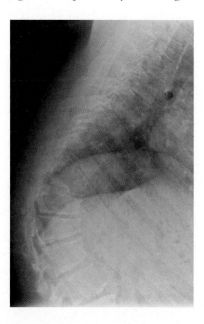

A. Disc space widening
B. Anterior wedging of at least four consecutive vertebral bodies
C. Decreased AP diameter of the vertebral bodies
D. Schmorl nodes

12 A 69-year-old female presents with neck pain and limited mobility. What is the most likely diagnosis?

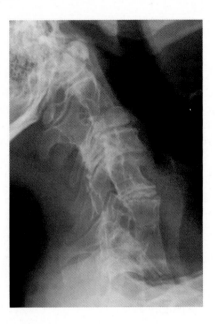

   A. Juvenile idiopathic arthritis
   B. Sprengel deformity
   C. Klippel-Feil syndrome
   D. Prior surgical fusion

13 A patient presents with chronic elbow pain. How is congenital dislocation of the radial head distinguished from a prior traumatic radial head dislocation?

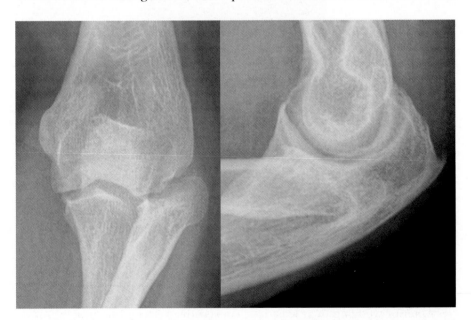

   A. The trochlea is dysplastic with congenital dislocation of the radial head.
   B. There is a fracture line in the radial head with congenital dislocation of the radial head.
   C. There is a persistent effusion associated with congenital dislocation of the radial head.
   D. The radial head is overgrown and dysplastic in congenital dislocation of the radial head.

14 A 10-year-old female presents with the image below. This patient most likely has which type of this disease?

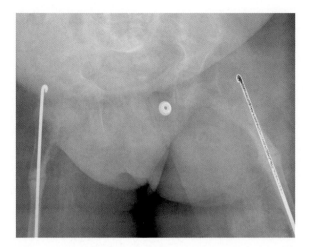

A. Type I
B. Type II
C. Type III
D. Type IV

15 A 78-year-old female presents with wrist pain. What is the most common location for the finding in the ulna?

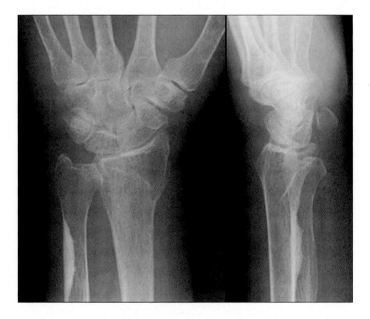

A. Upper extremity
B. Lower extremity
C. Spine
D. Skull

16 Which of the following statements about the movement of an os odontoideum on flexion and extension views is correct?

A. It moves with the atlas on flexion but not extension.
B. It moves with the axis on flexion but not extension.
C. It moves with the atlas on flexion and extension.
D. It moves with the axis on flexion and extension.

17 What is the primary etiology leading to the entity depicted in this pelvis radiograph?

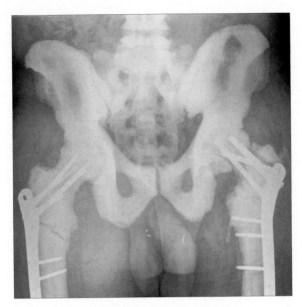

A. Abnormal osteoclast function
B. Abnormal osteoblast function
C. Abnormal calcium distribution
D. Abnormal phosphate distribution

18 A 38-year-old female presents with back pain. The finding at L4 most likely represents which of the below options?

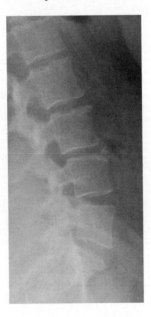

A. Syndesmophyte
B. Compression fracture
C. Gibbus deformity
D. Limbus vertebra

19 A 20-year-old male presents with scoliosis, as noted in the image below. What is the most common cause of scoliosis?

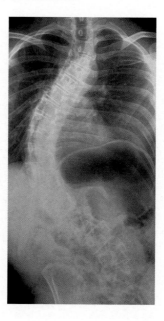

A. Idiopathic
B. Trauma
C. Leg length discrepancy
D. Congenital

20 A 17-year-old female presents with left hip pain resulting from developmental dysplasia of the hip. Which of the following radiographic findings is consistent with developmental dysplasia of the hip?

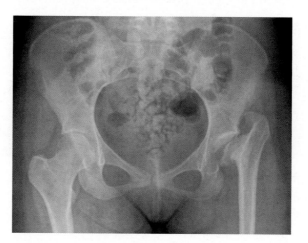

A. Downturning of the lateral acetabular roof
B. Coxa magna
C. Distal displacement of the trochanters
D. Anteversion of the acetabulum

21   An 18-month-old presents with scoliosis. Based on the three consecutive sagittal T2-weighted fat-saturation images, what is the most likely cause of scoliosis in this patient?

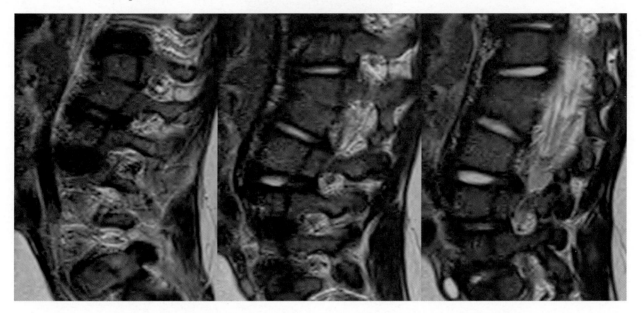

A. Trapezoidal vertebra
B. Neurofibromatosis type 1
C. Idiopathic
D. Hemivertebra

22   A 54-year-old male presents with knee pain. How many consecutive sagittal MR images, assuming a 5-mm-thick sagittal section, are required to make the diagnosis noted on the sagittal proton density images below?

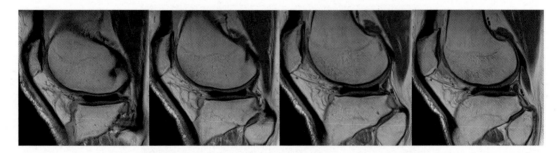

A. 2 or more
B. 3 or more
C. 4 or more
D. 5 or more

ANSWERS AND EXPLANATIONS

1 **Answer C.** Köhler disease is an osteochondrosis of the navicular of the foot. Similarly, Freiberg infraction is an osteochondrosis of the second metatarsal head. Patients with Köhler disease usually present at a young age with pain and swelling. Males are more commonly affected than are females. Radiographs demonstrate a sclerotic, flattened, and fragmented navicular.

Reference: Berquist T. *Musculoskeletal Imaging Companion.* 2nd ed. Philadelphia, PA: Lippincott Williams & Wilkins; 2007:435.

2 **Answer C.** Lunotriquetral carpal coalition is a common anatomic variant, present in roughly 0.1% of the population.

Reference: Timins ME. Osseous anatomic variants of the wrist: findings on MR imaging. *AJR Am J Roentgenol.* 1999;173(2):339–344.

3 **Answer D.** Images depict a shortened distal radius, which demonstrates abnormal ulnar tilt of its distal articular surface. Findings are characteristic of the Madelung deformity. Madelung deformity is often idiopathic but can also be seen in the setting of prior trauma, Turner disease, or skeletal dysplasias such as hereditary multiple exostoses. Scapholunate advanced collapse (SLAC wrist) is a pattern of wrist malalignment characterized by widening of the scapholunate interval, midcarpal collapse, proximal migration of the capitate, and radioscaphoid degenerative changes. Common causes of SLAC wrist include prior trauma or Calcium pyrophosphate deposition disease (CPPD) arthropathy. Kienböck disease describes a condition characterized by osteonecrosis of the lunate.

Reference: Manaster BJ, Roberts CC, Petersilge CA, et al. *Diagnostic Imaging: Musculoskeletal: Non-Traumatic Disease.* Manitoba, Canada: Amirsys; 2010;4:22–25.

4 **Answer A.** Plexiform neurofibromas would be most typical of neurofibromatosis type 1. Neurofibromatosis type 2 is characterized by multiple meningiomas, schwannomas, and ependymomas, but rarely true neurofibromas. Sturge-Weber and tuberous sclerosis are both neurocutaneous syndromes but are not associated with neurofibromas.

References: Korf BR. Plexiform neurofibromas. *Am J Med Genet.* 1999;89(1):31–37.
Manaster BJ, Roberts CC, Petersilge CA, et al. *Diagnostic Imaging: Musculoskeletal: Non-Traumatic Disease.* Manitoba, Canada: Amirsys; 2010;4:8–13.

5a **Answer A.** The radiograph demonstrates bilateral, bipartite patellae. Bipartite patella is a congenital/developmental variant, which can be painful, depending on the degree of abnormal motion at the synchondrosis. As seen in this radiograph, the accessory ossicle is usually located in the superolateral patella. Frequently, this abnormality is bilateral, as seen in this patient. Patients most commonly present with anterior knee pain.

References: Kavanagh EC, Zoga A, Omar I, et al. MRI findings in bipartite patella. *Skeletal Radiol.* 2007;36(3):209–214.
Keats TE, Anderson MW. *Atlas of Normal Roentgen Variants That May Simulate Disease.* 8th ed. Philadelphia, PA: Mosby; 2006:756.

5b **Answer C.** In a study of patients with anterior knee pain, the most common MRI finding was that of bone edema, hyperintense signal on T2-weighted fat saturated images, in the bipartite fragment. Sixty-six percent of patients had bone edema, and in 49% of patients, bone edema in the bipartite fragment was the only abnormal MRI finding.

Reference: Kavanagh EC, Zoga A, Omar I, et al. MRI findings in bipartite patella. *Skeletal Radiol.* 2007;36(3):209–214.

6 **Answer B.**   The classic syndrome depicted by the CT and radiograph is nail–patella syndrome. This autosomal dominant disorder has a clinical tetrad that includes the development of iliac horns, in conjunction with involvement of the nails, patella, and elbows. The iliac horns are pathognomonic for this condition; however, the nail changes are the most frequently encountered finding. The nail changes can be variable, and nails may be absent, hypoplastic, or dystrophic. The patella may be hypoplastic, misshapen, or absent. The typical elbow findings include a dysplastic radial head, hypoplastic capitellum and lateral epicondyle, and a prominent medial epicondyle.

References: Guidera KJ, Satterwhite Y, Ogden JA, et al. Nail patella syndrome: a review of 44 orthopaedic patients. *J Pediatr Orthop.* 1991;11:737–742.

Sweeney E, Fryer A, Mountford R, et al. Nail patella syndrome: a review of the phenotype aided by developmental biology. *J Med Genet.* 2003;40:153–162.

7 **Answer A.**   The image demonstrates acroosteolysis of multiple distal phalanges bilaterally. The differential for acroosteolysis includes resorptive, vascular, traumatic, inflammatory, infectious, and congenital etiologies. The resorptive causes include hyperparathyroidism and progressive systemic sclerosis. The vascular causes include frostbite, vasculitis, diabetes, meningococcemia, and amniotic band syndrome. The traumatic etiologies include burns, congenital insensitivity to pain, and occupational issues such as polyvinylchloride (PVC) workers and guitar players. The inflammatory causes include psoriatic arthritis and multicentric reticulohistiocytosis. Infectious causes include leprosy. Congenital etiologies include pycnodysostosis, Hajdu-Cheney syndrome, and Lesch-Nyhan syndrome.

Reference: Manaster BJ, Roberts CC, Petersilge CA, et al. *Diagnostic Imaging: Musculoskeletal: Non-Traumatic Disease.* Manitoba, Canada: Amirsys; 2010:6:6–9.

8 **Answer B.**   Fibrodysplasia ossificans progressiva, also known as myositis ossificans progressiva, is a hereditary disorder leading to mature ossification within soft tissues. This causes osseous bridging between osseous structures. The initial site of osseous bridging is typically the sternocleidomastoid followed by the shoulder girdle, upper arms, spine and pelvis. The pattern of ossification follows that of myositis ossificans in that initially there is a mass with edema distorting the fat planes, followed by ossification over the ensuing weeks and months. The disease is autosomal dominant, and the age of onset is approximately 5 years.

Reference: Manaster BJ, Roberts CC, Petersilge CA, et al. *Diagnostic Imaging: Musculoskeletal: Non-Traumatic Disease.* Manitoba, Canada: Amirsys; 2010:4:6.

9 **Answer C.**   Macrodystrophia lipomatosa is also called focal gigantism, nerve territory oriented macrodactyly, and neural fibrolipoma with macrodactyly. This is most commonly associated with lipomatosis of a nerve, typically the median nerve in the hand or the plantar nerve in the foot. By imaging, the disease presents as enlargement of a single or multiple digits, enlargement of the soft tissues, long and broad phalanges, splayed distal tufts, early osteoarthritis, and bowing deformities. In the hand, the second and third digits are most commonly affected. Scleroderma and leprosy would present with acroosteolysis. Scleroderma and dermatomyositis are often associated with soft tissue calcifications.

Reference: Manaster BJ, Roberts CC, Petersilge CA, et al. *Diagnostic Imaging: Musculoskeletal: Non-Traumatic Disease.* Manitoba, Canada: Amirsys; 2010:4:26–29.

10 **Answer B.**   Primary hypertrophic osteoarthropathy is also known as pachydermoperiostosis. Primary hypertrophic osteoarthropathy represents approximately 3% of cases of hypertrophic osteoarthropathy while secondary forms make up the remaining 97%. The most common cause of secondary hypertrophic osteoarthropathy is malignancy, accounting for approximately 90% of cases. Involvement of the tufts is not common in either primary or secondary cases; however, when it does occur, acroosteolysis is more commonly associated with primary hypertrophic osteoarthropathy while tuft hypertrophy is more commonly associated with secondary hypertrophic osteoarthropathy.

Reference: Manaster BJ, Roberts CC, Petersilge CA, et al. *Diagnostic Imaging: Musculoskeletal: Non-Traumatic Disease.* Manitoba, Canada: Amirsys; 2010:1:162–167.

[handwritten margin note: 1° = acro-osteo-lysis   2° = hypertrophy   Think 1° comes before 2° and a comes before h]

11   **Answer D.**   The image demonstrates the classic findings of Scheuermann disease. These findings include decreased disc space heights, increased AP diameter of the involved vertebral bodies, anterior wedging of at least 5 degrees involving three or more consecutive vertebral bodies, and Schmorl nodes. A Schmorl node most commonly results from intraosseous disc herniation through a weakened vertebral endplate.

Reference: Chew FS. *The Core Curriculum: Musculoskeletal Imaging.* Philadelphia, PA: Lippincott Williams & Wilkins; 2003:453.

12   **Answer C.**   The image depicts Klippel-Feil syndrome, which is failure of cervical segmentation at multiple levels. This is often associated with a short neck and a low hairline. These patients have limited cervical motion as well as an increased risk for renal; spinal cord; and inner-, middle-, and outer-ear abnormalities. This syndrome can be differentiated from surgical fusion by the narrow AP dimension of the vertebral bodies, as is seen in the lower cervical spine in this case. Juvenile idiopathic arthritis, which has a similar appearance, typically involves more levels. Sprengel deformity is seen in one-third of patients with Klippel-Feil syndrome and is tethering of the scapula to the cervical spine by a fibrous band, resulting in a high position of the scapula.

Reference: Manaster BJ, May DA, Disler DG. *The Requisites: Musculoskeletal Imaging.* 3rd ed. Philadelphia, PA: Mosby; 2007:594–595.

13   **Answer D.**   The images demonstrate a case of congenital dislocation of the radial head. This entity can be distinguished from a postnatal dislocation of the radial head by overgrowth and dysplasia of the radial head. There may also be a dysplastic configuration of the capitellum.

Reference: Manaster BJ, May DA, Disler DG. *The Requisites: Musculoskeletal Imaging.* 3rd ed. Philadelphia, PA: Mosby; 2007:121–122.

14   **Answer C.**   The radiograph is of a 10-year-old female with osteogenesis imperfecta. There are four types. Type I is the least severe and has gracile, thin tubular bones and osteopenia. Type II is the most severe and is typically lethal at the time of or shortly after birth. Type III is the most severe form that survives into childhood and adulthood. It is the most likely form to be radiographed for fractures. In this form the bones are short and thick and often have multiple fractures with hypertrophic callus, the fractures are subject to nonunion or malunion, and the bones may suffer bowing deformities. Type IV is similar to Type I, except Type IV is more likely to have basilar skull impression. Type I is the most common, Type II is the second most common, Type III is the third most common, and finally Type IV is the least common. Osteogenesis imperfecta is the result of a genetic defect in collagen.

Reference: Manaster BJ, Roberts CC, Petersilge CA, et al. *Diagnostic Imaging: Musculoskeletal: Non-Traumatic Disease.* Manitoba, Canada: Amirsys; 2010:4:14–19.

15   **Answer B.**   The images of the wrist depict melorheostosis, which has the appearance of dripping candle wax. This is often the result of hyperostosis that is mostly periosteal but may also be endosteal with intramedullary extension. It may also appear as linear intraosseous sclerosis, as rounded osteoma-like foci or sclerosis, or less commonly as soft tissue masses. This may occur in a single bone or in multiple bones in an extremity in a sclerotomal distribution. The most common location is the lower extremity. It may rarely occur in the spine, but it typically spares the skull and facial bones.

Reference: Manaster BJ, Roberts CC, Petersilge CA, et al. *Diagnostic Imaging: Musculoskeletal: Non-Traumatic Disease*. Manitoba, Canada: Amirsys; 2010:5:34–37.

16   **Answer C.**   The os odontoideum is a large ossicle that lies in the space normally occupied by the odontoid process. It is separated from the hypoplastic odontoid by a gap. Its appearance may simulate a fracture. The os odontoideum is fixed to the arch of the atlas and moves with it on flexion and extension views.

Reference: Manaster BJ, May DA, Disler DG. *The Requisites: Musculoskeletal Imaging*. 3rd ed. Philadelphia, PA: Mosby; 2007:166–168.

17   **Answer A.**   The pelvis radiograph depicts osteopetrosis, as noted by the diffusely dense bones. This results from abnormal osteoclast function. The abnormal osteoclasts lead to an imbalance between bone formation and bone resorption. The bone is unable to be remodeled appropriately, and a normal intramedullary space is not created. Bone production is, however, not impaired. Collectively, this results in a predisposition to fractures at sites of stress and subsequent poor fracture healing. Radiographically, the bones are diffusely and uniformly dense with loss of the normal corticomedullary differentiation. It involves the epiphysis, metaphysis, and diaphysis. There is undertubulation of the metaphysis, often seen in the distal femur. The cranial vault may be diffusely thickened and sclerotic with loss of the diploic space. There may be sclerosis of the skull base. The spine may have a bone-within-a-bone appearance.

Reference: Manaster BJ, Roberts CC, Petersilge CA, et al. *Diagnostic Imaging: Musculoskeletal: Non-Traumatic Disease*. Manitoba, Canada: Amirsys; 2010:5:42–47.

18   **Answer D.**   The finding at L4 is a limbus vertebra. This typically results from an intraosseous herniation in the growing spine that may separate the ring apophysis from the vertebral body. It is seen on a lateral radiograph as a triangular ossicle, most commonly located at the anterior–superior border of the vertebral body. Limbus vertebra can be confused with vertebral body fractures; however, their characteristic appearance should allow for differentiation from a fracture. A gibbus deformity is an acute kyphosis seen in association with Pott disease, which is related to tuberculosis infection of the spine. Syndesmophytes are thin vertical ossifications in the annulus fibrosis at the discovertebral junction. These are commonly seen in association with ankylosing spondylitis.

Reference: Manaster BJ, May DA, Disler DG. *The Requisites: Musculoskeletal Imaging*. 3rd ed. Philadelphia, PA: Mosby; 2007:310–311.

19   **Answer A.**   The most common cause of scoliosis is idiopathic, accounting for approximately 85% of cases. Other causes of scoliosis include leg length discrepancy, congenital causes, neuromuscular causes, neurofibromatosis, connective tissue disorders, trauma, tumors, and radiation therapy.

Reference: Manaster BJ, May DA, Disler DG. *The Requisites: Musculoskeletal Imaging*. 3rd ed. Philadelphia, PA: Mosby; 2007:582–589.

20   **Answer B.**   Coxa magna represents a broadened femoral head with a short and wide femoral neck. This is seen in developmental dysplasia of the hip (DDH). Coxa magna results in femoral shortening, which leads to proximal displacement of both the lesser and greater trochanters. The least severe acetabular change is upturning of the lateral acetabular roof. The most severe acetabular change is lack of formation of the acetabulum with the femoral head forming a pseudoarticulation with the iliac bone. The acetabulum is retroverted in 37% of cases. DDH is bilateral in 20% of cases; therefore, the contralateral hip should be imaged. In infants, imaging of DDH is performed with ultrasound to avoid radiation.

Reference: Manaster BJ, Roberts CC, Petersilge CA, et al. *Diagnostic Imaging: Musculoskeletal: Non-Traumatic Disease.* Manitoba, Canada: Amirsys; 2010:4:30–35.

21 Answer D.   Between L1 and L2, a hemivertebra is noted. Two pedicles are noted on the first two images; however, on the third image, there is the appearance of one enlarged vertebral body. This represents the native L2 vertebral body and the hemivertebra adjacent to it without an intervening disc. Only one pedicle was noted on the contralateral side, which is not shown on the provided images.

References: Chew FS. *The Core Curriculum: Musculoskeletal Imaging.* Philadelphia, PA: Lippincott Williams & Wilkins; 2003:452–453.
Manaster BJ, May DA, Disler DG. *The Requisites: Musculoskeletal Imaging.* 3rd ed. Philadelphia, PA: Mosby; 2007:582–585.

22 Answer B.   The images of the lateral meniscus demonstrate the bow tie appearance of the lateral meniscus on four consecutive sagittal images. To make the diagnosis of a discoid meniscus, the bow tie appearance should be present on at least three consecutive sagittal images, assuming 5-mm-thick sagittal sections. On coronal images, the diagnosis may be made if the meniscus, from the free edge margin to the periphery of the body of the meniscus, measures >1.4 cm. The presence of a discoid meniscus is important because it may be the source of pain or locking even in the absence of a tear. It also is more likely to tear due to its altered biomechanical properties. It has been estimated that 2.7% of the population may have a discoid meniscus. They are more common in the lateral meniscus but may occur in the medial meniscus or both the medial and lateral meniscus in the same knee or may be bilateral. They are more frequently found in males.

References: Manaster BJ, May DA, Disler DG. *The Requisites: Musculoskeletal Imaging.* 3rd ed. Philadelphia, PA: Mosby; 2007:230–232.
Resnick D, Kang HS, Pretterklieber ML. *Internal Derangements of Joints.* 2nd ed. Philadelphia, PA: Saunders; 2007:1689–1697.

1   A 63-year-old paraplegic male is imaged. A right hip radiograph and CT from
    3 years prior are presented for comparison to the current CT of the right hip.
    What is the most likely diagnosis?

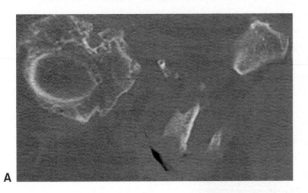

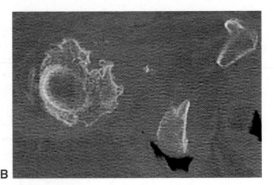

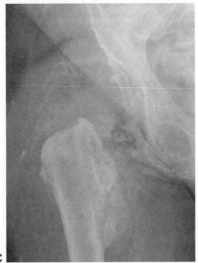

A. Current **B.** 3 years prior **C.** 3 years prior

A. Soft tissue abscess
B. Joint effusion
C. Chronic osteomyelitis
D. Myositis

2a A 26-year-old male is transferred from an outside institution after a radiograph at that institution was interpreted as a possible malignancy of the right femur. Based on the radiographs below, what is the most likely diagnosis?

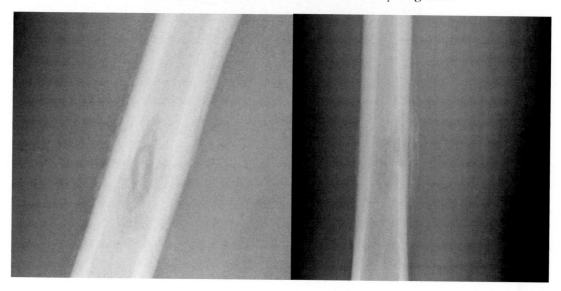

    A. Osteosarcoma
    B. Ewing sarcoma
    C. Metastatic disease
    D. Osteomyelitis

2b A CT examination of the previous finding was performed. What is indicated by the arrow in the coronal CT image below performed in bone window?

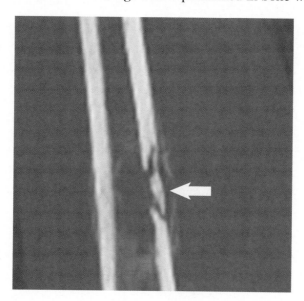

    A. Sequestrum
    B. Involucrum
    C. Periosteal reaction
    D. Sinus tract

2c   An MRI of the above finding was performed. What is indicated by the arrow on the axial T1 fat-saturated postcontrast image below?

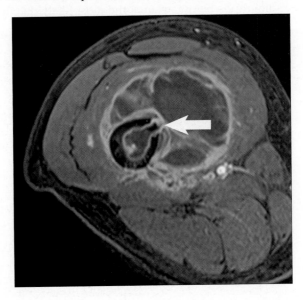

A. Sequestrum
B. Involucrum
C. Cloaca
D. Periosteum

3   Pictured below are two radiographs of a diabetic right foot, one current and one 6 months prior immediately after amputation of a portion of the great toe. In diabetic patients, what is the most common site of osteomyelitis of the foot?

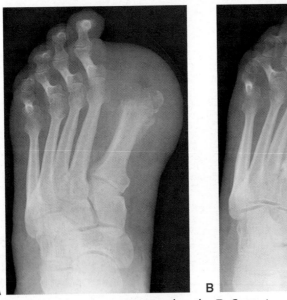
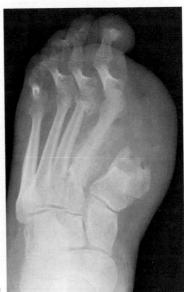

A   B

A. 6 months prior **B.** Current

A. Navicular and medial cuneiform
B. Third and fourth metatarsal shafts
C. Cuboid and lateral cuneiform
D. First and fifth metatarsal heads

4   A 7-year-old female presents to the emergency department with ankle swelling. MR images of the distal tibial and fibular metaphyses are presented. What is the most likely diagnosis?

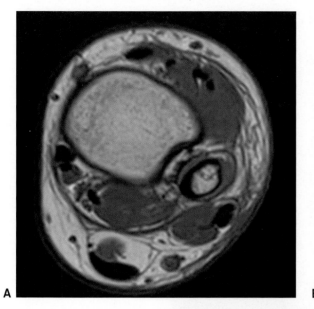

A

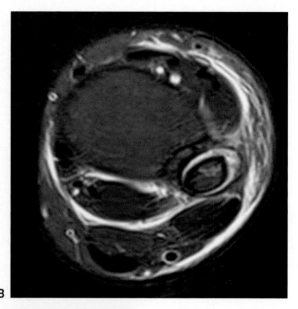

B

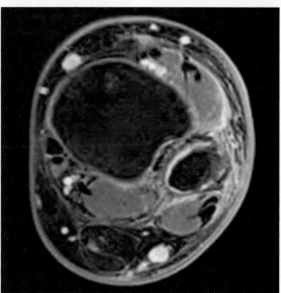

C

A. Axial T1 weighted **B.** Axial T2 weighted fat saturated **C.** Axial T1 weighted fat saturated postcontrast

   A. Necrotizing fasciitis
   B. Subperiosteal abscess
   C. Pyomyositis
   D. Gas gangrene

5   Images of the fifth metatarsal–phalangeal joint are presented in a 49-year-old patient. Which of the following is the earliest radiographic finding of septic arthritis?

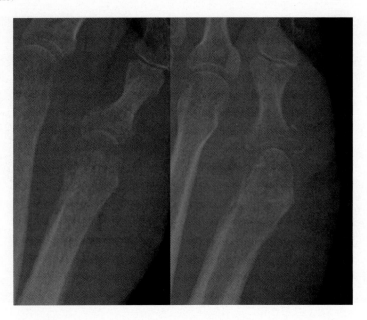

A. Osteomyelitis
B. Joint effusion
C. Periarticular osteoporosis
D. Erosions

6   A 25-year-old male presents to the emergency department complaining of left hip pain. Based on the MR images below, what is the diagnosis?

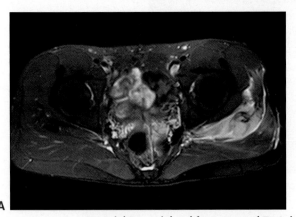
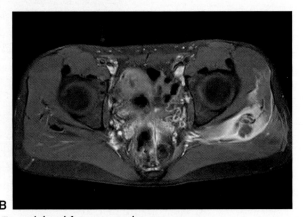

A   B

A. Axial T2 weighted fat saturated **B.** Axial T1 weighted fat saturated postcontrast

A. Cellulitis
B. Pyomyositis
C. Osteomyelitis
D. Necrotizing fasciitis

7   Presented below are two MR images of osteomyelitis of the second metatarsal in a diabetic patient. Which T1-weighted signal pattern is most reliable in diagnosing osteomyelitis of the foot?

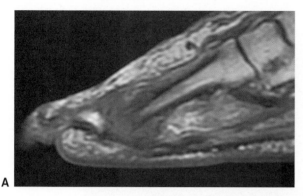 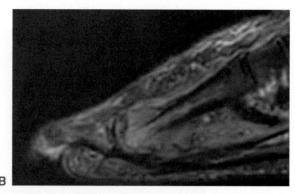

A **A.** Sagittal T1 weighted **B.** Sagittal T2 weighted fat saturated

A. Low geographic, medullary T1 signal
B. Low hazy, reticulated T1 signal
C. Low subcortical T1 signal
D. Low subchondral T1 signal

8   A 24-year-old female presents with swelling of the elbow and forearm. What is the characteristic appearance of the fibrous capsule of an abscess on MRI?

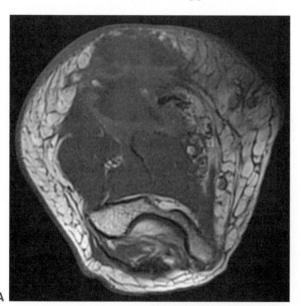 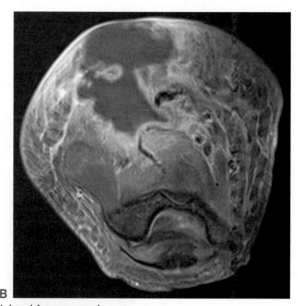

A **A.** Axial T1 weighted **B.** Axial T1 weighted fat saturated postcontrast

A. Thin, nonenhancing
B. Thin, enhancing
C. Thick, nonenhancing
D. Thick, enhancing

9 A 65-year-old male presents to the emergency room with a fever, malaise, and bilateral posterior thigh pain. A CT of the bilateral lower extremities was performed. Which of the following microorganisms is most often implicated in the condition depicted on the CT image?

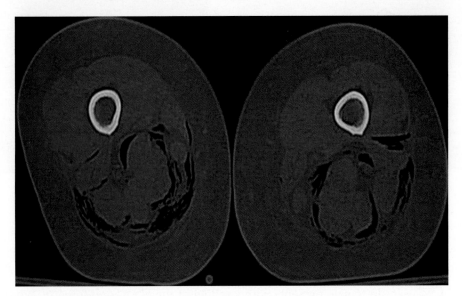

A. *Salmonella*
B. *Staphylococcus*
C. *Streptococcus*
D. Polymicrobial

10a A 59-year-old diabetic male presents with the following images of the right foot. What is the earliest osseous radiographic sign of osteomyelitis?

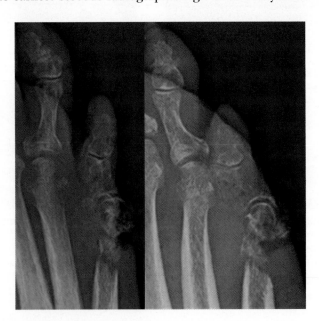

A. Permeative osseous destruction
B. Endosteal scalloping
C. Indistinctness of the cortex
D. Periosteal reaction

10b The ordering physician is concerned about gangrene of the foot. Which of the following MRI findings is most critical in diagnosing gangrene of the foot?

    A. Signal voids resulting from gas created by gas-forming organisms
    B. Skin thickening and cellulitis
    C. Areas of absent contrast enhancement
    D. Areas of associated osteomyelitis

11 A 54-year-old diabetic male presents with the images below. Which MRI finding is typically present in cellulitis and not present in soft tissue edema associated with diabetic vasculopathy?

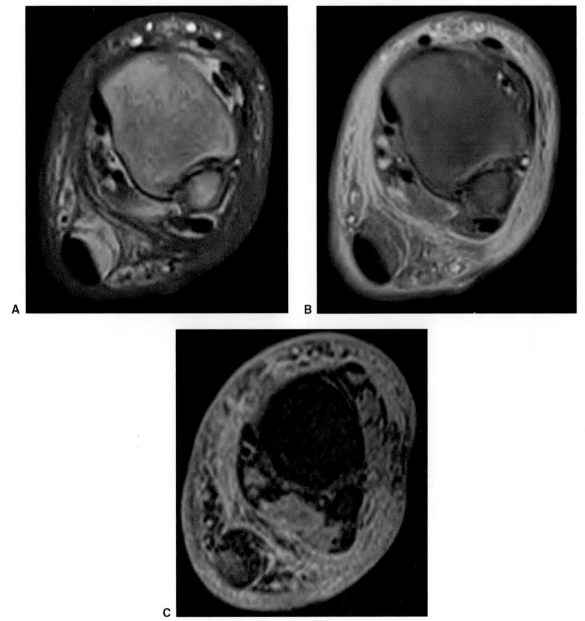

A. Axial T1 weighted **B.** Axial T2 weighted fat saturated **C.** Axial T1 weighted fat saturated postcontrast

    A. Contrast enhancement of the involved area.
    B. T1-weighted signal of the affected area is hypointense to fat.
    C. T2-weighted signal of the affected area is hyperintense to muscle.
    D. A skin ulceration is present in the affected area.

12 A 34-year-old diabetic male with a known neuropathic midfoot presents with the MR images below. Which of the following MRI features suggests superimposed osteomyelitis in a neuropathic foot?

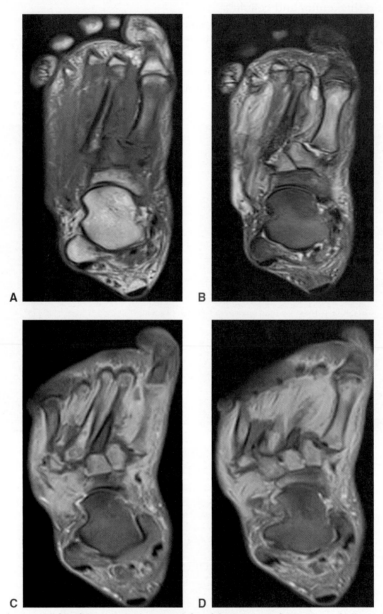

A. Long axis T1 weighted **B.** Long axis T2 weighted fat saturated **C.** Long axis T1 weighted fat saturated postcontrast **D.** Long axis T1 weighted fat saturated postcontrast

    A. Intra-articular loose bodies
    B. Subchondral cystic change
    C. Thin rim enhancement of joint effusions
    D. Soft tissue abscess

ANSWERS AND EXPLANATIONS

1 **Answer C.** This case is of a paraplegic male with chronic decubitus ulcers, as noted by the air adjacent to the ischium on both the CT and radiograph images. This case represents chronic osteomyelitis. In the interval from the prior study, ischial changes include increased osseous destruction, sclerosis, and thickening of the remaining cortex consistent with chronic osteomyelitis. Other findings that can be seen with chronic osteomyelitis include periosteal new bone formation, sequestrum and involucrum formation, cloaca formation, and sinus tracts to the skin surface. Chronic osteomyelitis has been associated with development of squamous cell carcinoma within sinus tracts in 0.2% to 1.6% of patients.

References: Manaster BJ, Roberts CC, Petersilge CA, et al. *Diagnostic Imaging: Musculoskeletal: Non-Traumatic Disease.* Manitoba, Canada: Amirsys; 2010:8:18–21.
Weissman BN. *Imaging of Arthritis and Metabolic Bone Disease.* Philadelphia, PA: Saunders; 2009:322.

2a **Answer D.** The radiographs depict a sequestrum associated with osteomyelitis. The appearance is not typical for osteosarcoma, Ewing sarcoma, or metastatic disease, and the age is also not typical for Ewing sarcoma. 80% to 90% of patients diagnosed with Ewing sarcoma are 20 years of age or younger. After further inquiry, the patient admitted to recent IV drug use.

References: Manaster BJ, Roberts CC, Petersilge CA, et al. *Diagnostic Imaging: Musculoskeletal: Non-Traumatic Disease.* Manitoba, Canada: Amirsys; 2010:8:6–11.
Weissman BN. *Imaging of Arthritis and Metabolic Bone Disease.* Philadelphia, PA: Saunders; 2009:314–318.

2b **Answer A.** The coronal CT image depicts a sequestrum, which is necrotic bone surrounded by purulent material or granulation tissue. The sequestrum is usually of normal density and may harbor bacteria serving as a source for chronic osteomyelitis. The sequestrum and purulent material are typically surrounded by a bone shell called the involucrum, which is also seen in this image surrounding the sequestrum. Periosteal reaction and sinus tracts may be associated with osteomyelitis as well.

References: Manaster BJ, Roberts CC, Petersilge CA, et al. *Diagnostic Imaging: Musculoskeletal: Non-Traumatic Disease.* Manitoba, Canada: Amirsys; 2010:8:6–11.
Weissman BN. *Imaging of Arthritis and Metabolic Bone Disease.* Philadelphia, PA: Saunders; 2009:314–318.

2c **Answer C.** The arrow points to the cloaca, which is a cortical and periosteal defect that allows pus to drain from the infected medullary cavity into the adjacent surrounded tissues. This can lead to abscess formation, which is seen in this case.

References: Manaster BJ, Roberts CC, Petersilge CA, et al. *Diagnostic Imaging: Musculoskeletal: Non-Traumatic Disease.* Manitoba, Canada: Amirsys; 2010:8:6–11.
Weissman BN. *Imaging of Arthritis and Metabolic Bone Disease.* Philadelphia, PA: Saunders; 2009:314–318.

3 **Answer D.** Osteomyelitis typically occurs at sites of increased pressure. In the foot, the most common sites are the first and fifth metatarsal heads, the phalanges, and the calcaneus. In this case, the original image demonstrated osteomyelitis of the first metatarsal head. Six months later, after resection of the first metatarsal head, the second metatarsal demonstrates osteomyelitis.

Reference: Weissman BN. *Imaging of Arthritis and Metabolic Bone Disease.* Philadelphia, PA: Saunders; 2009:326.

4   **Answer B.**   The images demonstrate a subperiosteal abscess of the distal fibular metaphysis. In children, relative to adults, the periosteum is more loosely attached to the cortex. As pus develops in the medullary space it eventually breaks through the cortex and fills the subperiosteal space, creating a subperiosteal abscess. The most common infectious etiology is *S. aureus*.

References: Manaster BJ, Roberts CC, Petersilge CA, et al. *Diagnostic Imaging: Musculoskeletal: Non-Traumatic Disease*. Manitoba, Canada: Amirsys; 2010:8:2–5.
Weissman BN. *Imaging of Arthritis and Metabolic Bone Disease*. Philadelphia, PA: Saunders; 2009:328–330.

5   **Answer B.**   The earliest radiographic sign of a septic joint is a joint effusion. Later findings include periarticular osteoporosis, cartilage destruction seen as joint space narrowing, indistinctness of the cortical bone, marginal erosions, osteomyelitis, sclerosis, and eventually ankylosis.

References: Manaster BJ, Roberts CC, Petersilge CA, et al. *Diagnostic Imaging: Musculoskeletal: Non-Traumatic Disease*. Manitoba, Canada: Amirsys; 2010:8:22–27.
Weissman BN. *Imaging of Arthritis and Metabolic Bone Disease*. Philadelphia, PA: Saunders; 2009:330.

6   **Answer B.**   The images note pyomyositis of the gluteal musculature in the setting of IV drug abuse. There is a component of cellulitis as well, but this is not the predominant finding. Pyomyositis is demonstrated by an intramuscular abscess with an enhancing peripheral rim. There is typically inflammation in the adjacent soft tissues. No changes are noted in the bone marrow signal to suggest osteomyelitis. There is no enhancement of the deep fascia to suggest necrotizing fasciitis.

References: Manaster BJ, Roberts CC, Petersilge CA, et al. *Diagnostic Imaging: Musculoskeletal: Non-Traumatic Disease*. Manitoba, Canada: Amirsys; 2010:8:30–33.
Weissman BN. *Imaging of Arthritis and Metabolic Bone Disease*. Philadelphia, PA: Saunders; 2009:333–334.

7   **Answer A.**   The most reliable T1-weighted MR signal pattern of pedal osteomyelitis is low signal in a geographic medullary distribution. In the study by Collins MS et al, 100% of the surgically proven cases of osteomyelitis had this T1 signal pattern with corresponding high signal on T2-weighted fat-saturated images. If the T1 signal pattern did not match a geographic medullary pattern, the authors of this paper excluded the diagnosis of osteomyelitis. The other T1 signal patterns provided as answer options do not represent true cases of osteomyelitis, but may be seen in cases of reactive edema.

References: Collins MS, Schaar MM, Wenger DE, et al. T1 weighted MRI characteristics of pedal osteomyelitis. *AJR Am J Roentgenol*. 2005;185:386–393.
Manaster BJ, Roberts CC, Petersilge CA, et al. *Diagnostic Imaging: Musculoskeletal: Non-Traumatic Disease*. Manitoba, Canada: Amirsys; 2010:8:6–11.

8   **Answer D.**   The fibrous capsule of a soft tissue abscess characteristically has a thick, enhancing rim. The abscess centrally has low T1-weighted and high T2-weighted signal. Other MRI findings that can be seen with a soft tissue abscess include cellulitis, fasciitis, myositis or pyomyositis, adjacent reactive bone formation or saucerization, or sinus tracts to the skin surface.

References: Manaster BJ, Roberts CC, Petersilge CA, et al. *Diagnostic Imaging: Musculoskeletal: Non-Traumatic Disease*. Manitoba, Canada: Amirsys; 2010:8:30–33.
Weissman BN. *Imaging of Arthritis and Metabolic Bone Disease*. Philadelphia, PA: Saunders; 2009:333.

9 **Answer D.** The majority of the cases of necrotizing fasciitis are caused by a polymicrobial infection, including the involvement of both aerobes and anaerobes, and are often seeded by an underlying preexisting infection. Approximately 15% of the cases of necrotizing fasciitis can be attributed to a single pathogen, and group A streptococci, previously coined "the flesh-eating bacteria" account for ~10% of these cases. The classic CT finding of necrotizing fasciitis is soft tissue gas associated with fluid collections within the deep fascial planes.

References: Fugitt JB, Puckett ML, Quigley MM, et al. Necrotizing fasciitis. *RadioGraphics.* 2004;24:1472–1476.

Mulcahy H, Richardson ML. Imaging of necrotizing fasciitis: self-assessment module. *AJR Am J Roentgenol.* 2010;195:S66–S69.

10a **Answer C.** Typically, radiographs do not demonstrate osseous changes during the first 1 to 2 weeks after the initiation of the infection. The earliest osseous change of osteomyelitis is indistinctness of the cortex. This is followed by permeative osseous destruction, endosteal scalloping, and periosteal reaction. Later changes include the formation of a sequestrum, an involucrum, or an abscess.

Manaster BJ, Roberts CC, Petersilge CA, et al. *Diagnostic Imaging: Musculoskeletal: Non-Traumatic Disease.* Manitoba, Canada: Amirsys; 2010:8:8–11.

10b **Answer C.** The most critical MRI finding in diagnosing gangrene of the foot is detecting areas of nonenhancement. This results from devitalization of the tissue. The skin may be focally thinned within the involved area. Gas may be present within the area involved; however, this is more commonly the result of an ulcer communicating with the skin surface than from gas from the infecting organism. Osteomyelitis may be an associated finding, but alone it does not make the diagnosis of gangrene.

Reference: Russell JM, Peterson JJ, Bancroft LW. MR imaging of the diabetic foot. *Magn Reson Imaging Clin N Am.* 2008;16:59–70.

11 **Answer A.** Cellulitis is differentiated from soft tissue edema in diabetic patients with vasculopathy by the intense soft tissue enhancement associated with cellulitis. Both cellulitis and edema will have T1 signal, which is hypointense to fat, and T2 signal, which is hyperintense to muscle. Ulceration is not required to make the diagnosis of cellulitis.

Reference: Russell JM, Peterson JJ, Bancroft LW. MR imaging of the diabetic foot. *Magn Reson Imaging Clin N Am.* 2008;16:59–70.

12 **Answer D.** Osteomyelitis superimposed on a neuropathic joint may be difficult to detect. There are, however, MRI signs that may suggest the presence of osteomyelitis in these cases. These include sinus tracts, replacement of the soft tissue fat, fluid collections, disappearance of subchondral cysts on sequential imaging, and extensive marrow abnormalities. Signs that suggest osteomyelitis is not present include thin rim enhancement of joint effusions, the presence of subchondral cysts, and the presence of intra-articular loose bodies. Features that can be seen in both osteomyelitis and neuropathic joints and, therefore, do not help distinguish the two include erosions, fragmentation, subluxations, and bone proliferations. In this case, there is a soft tissue abscess between the first and second metatarsal heads, diffuse replacement of the soft tissue fat, and extensive marrow abnormalities.

Reference: Russell JM, Peterson JJ, Bancroft LW. MR imaging of the diabetic foot. *Magn Reson Imaging Clin N Am.* 2008;16:59–70.

QUESTIONS

1 The distribution of skeletal lesions in Ollier disease is best described as

A. mostly involving the skull and spine.
B. predominantly unilateral or asymmetric.
C. greater involvement of diaphysis of the long bones when compared to metaphysis.
D. bilateral, symmetric epiphyseal involvement.

2 Ewing sarcoma characteristically occurs in which part of the bone?

A. Epiphysis
B. Metaphysis
C. Metadiaphysis
D. Periosteum

3 A 45-year-old male presents with painful foot nodules. Based on the MR images, what is the most likely diagnosis?

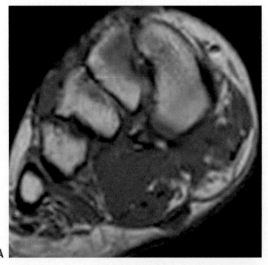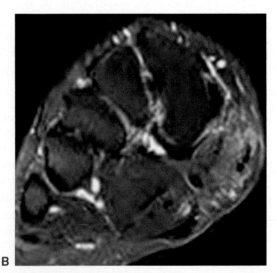

A. Short axis T1 weighted **B.** Short axis T2 weighted fat saturated

A. Forestier disease
B. Plantar fasciopathy
C. Plantar fibromatosis
D. Morton neuroma

4 A 45-year-old male presents to his primary care provider with a palpable mass. The patient was informed the mass is benign. In regard to the imaged pathology, which feature, when present, would be concerning for malignancy?

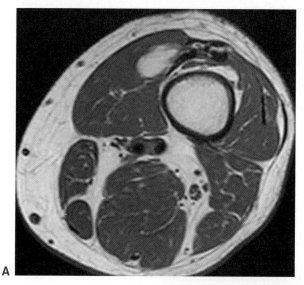 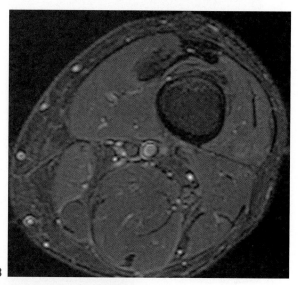

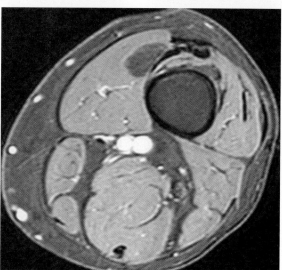

A. Axial T1 weighted **B.** Axial T2 weighted fat saturated **C.** Axial T1 weighted fat saturated postcontrast

A. Thin septations
B. Nonadipose components
C. Intramuscular involvement
D. Thin rim enhancement

5 What is the most frequent donor site for cancellous bone grafting?
A. Rib
B. Iliac crest
C. Fibula
D. Distal radius

6 Which of the following would be a primary differential consideration for the disease process depicted by the MR images?

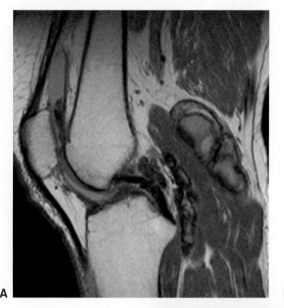
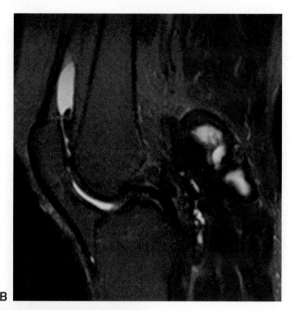
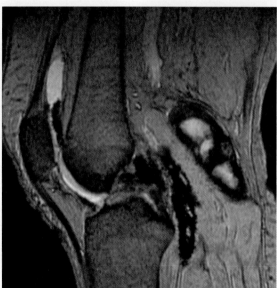

A. Sagittal proton density **B.** Sagittal T2 weighted fat saturated **C.** Sagittal T2* weighted gradient echo

A. Synovial chondromatosis
B. Pigmented villonodular synovitis
C. Amyloid arthropathy
D. Synovial cell sarcoma

7 A 30-year-old male presents with a lesion in the proximal tibia. It is described as a well-defined, lytic lesion without a defined sclerotic margin, eccentric in location, and extending to the subarticular margin of the tibia. What is the most likely diagnosis?

A. Osteosarcoma
B. Giant cell tumor
C. Ewing sarcoma
D. Metastasis

8   A 17-year-old female presented with leg swelling. Based on the images, what is the most likely diagnosis?

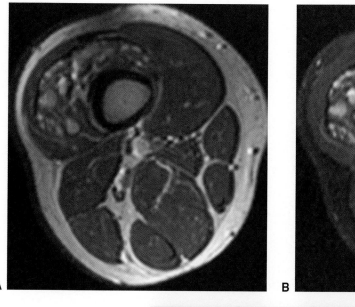
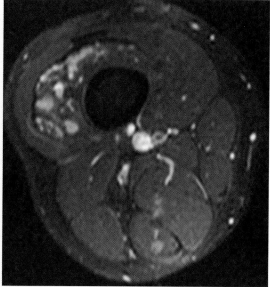
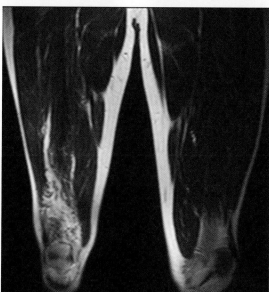

A. Axial T2 weighted **B.** Axial T1 weighted fat saturated postcontrast **C.** Coronal T1 weighted

    A. Intramuscular hemangioma
    B. Klippel-Trenaunay-Weber syndrome
    C. Arteriovascular malformation
    D. Pseudoaneurysm

9   Which of the following is an appropriate indication for treatment of a nonossifying fibroma?

    A. Pathologic fracture
    B. Size >3 cm
    C. Eccentric location
    D. Lucent radiographic appearance

10 A 60-year-old female patient had the following bone scan and radiograph. What is the most likely diagnosis?

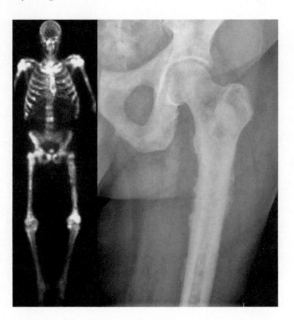

A. Paget disease
B. Multiple myeloma
C. Radiation osteitis
D. Osteoblastic metastases

11 A 6-year-old male presents to his pediatrician with a palpable lump involving his right lower leg. Based on the radiographs of his right tibia/fibula, which of the following is the most likely diagnosis?

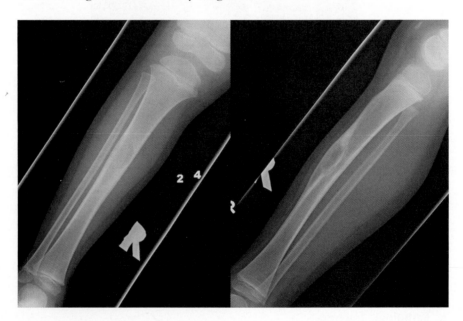

A. Aneurysmal bone cyst
B. Osteofibrous dysplasia
C. Lymphoma
D. Chondroblastoma

12 An 8-year-old girl presents with pain in the left hand fifth digit. There is no prior history of trauma. Which of the following is the most likely diagnosis?

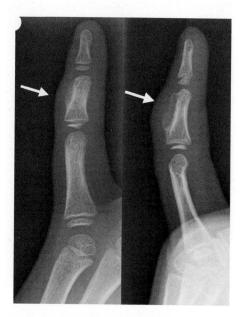

    A. Myositis ossificans
    B. Osteochondroma
    C. Osteosarcoma
    D. Bizarre parosteal osteochondromatous proliferation (BPOP)

13 Which of the following entities is seen in association with the tumor noted in the image below?

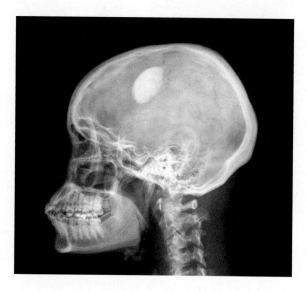

    A. Ollier disease
    B. Gardner syndrome
    C. Peutz Jeghers syndrome
    D. Maffucci syndrome

14 Regarding the disease process in the image below, which of the following statements best characterizes the potential for malignancy?

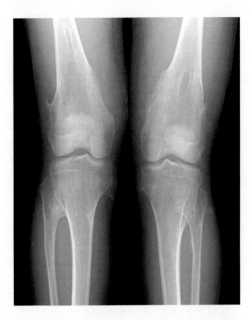

    A. The patient is at a higher risk for transformation to osteosarcoma.

    B. The patient is at a higher risk for osseous metastases to the lung.

    C. The patient is at a higher risk for osseous skip lesions within the affected bone.

    D. The patient is at a higher risk for transformation to chondrosarcoma.

15 A nerve sheath tumor is depicted in the images below. Which of the following statements about MR imaging signs of nerve sheath tumors is correct?

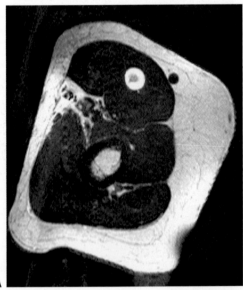 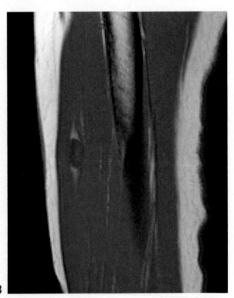

A. Axial T2 weighted **B.** Sagittal T1 weighted

    A. The fascicular sign is specific for a neurofibroma.

    B. The target sign demonstrates increased signal centrally and more intermediate signal seen in the periphery of the lesion on T2-weighted sequences.

    C. The split fat sign is specific for a neurofibroma.

    D. An eccentrically positioned lesion in relation to the parent nerve suggests a schwannoma.

16 Which of the following findings would suggest malignant transformation of an osteochondroma to a chondrosarcoma?

    A. Growth of a previously unchanged osteochondroma in a skeletally immature patient

    B. Thickening of the cartilaginous cap to >1.0 cm

    C. Development of a fluid signal intensity bursa overlying the lesion

    D. Focal lucencies of destruction in the interior of a lesion

17 Which of the following statements about the MRI appearance of synovial chondromatosis is correct?

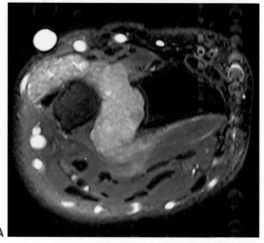 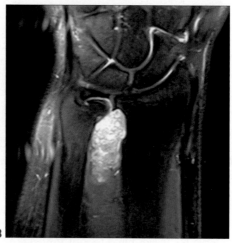

A. Axial T2 weighted fat saturated **B.** Coronal T2 weighted fat saturated

    A. The adjacent bone typically does not have evident erosions.

    B. It typically shows low MR signal and blooming artifact.

    C. The chondromatosis bodies are commonly low on T1 and high on T2.

    D. The involved synovium does not typically enhance.

18 Which of the following best characterizes the most common location for the lesion depicted in the image below?

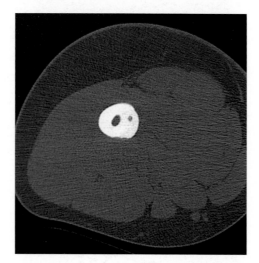

    A. The most common long bone to be involved is the femur.

    B. For intracapsular lesions, the most common location is the femoral condyle of the knee.

    C. Thoracic spine location is more common than the cervical or lumbar spine.

    D. An intramedullary location is more common than an intracortical location.

19 Which of the following is correct regarding the MRI appearance of synovial sarcoma?

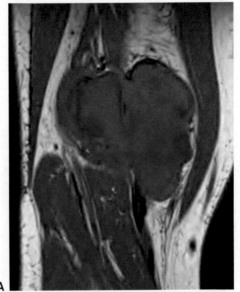 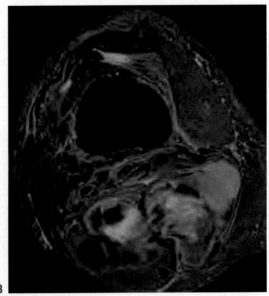

A. Coronal T1 **B.** Axial T2 fat saturated

A. The T1 appearance is typically hyperintense to muscle.
B. The enhancement is typically homogeneous.
C. It can have foci of low signal resulting from areas of mineralization.
D. The T2 appearance is typically isointense to muscle.

20 Regarding the lesion in the image below, which of the following best describes the most common location?

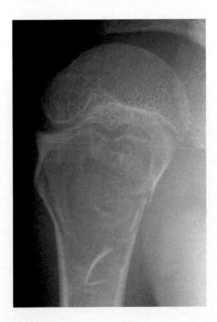

A. Intramedullary, central
B. Intracortical, central
C. Intramedullary, eccentric
D. Intracortical, eccentric

* **21** Which approach would be the most appropriate for percutaneous image-guided biopsy in this lesion?

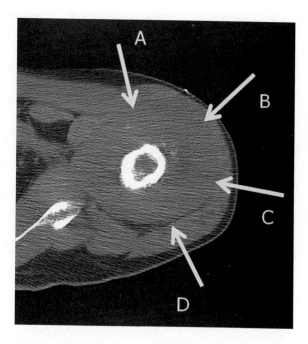

A. A
B. B
C. C
D. D

22 Regarding the lesion in the image below, which of the following represents the best management?

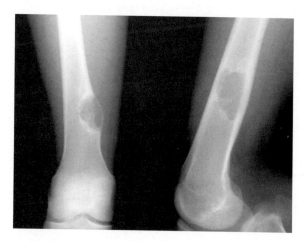

A. The lesion is benign and should be not be biopsied.
B. The lesion is indeterminate and should be biopsied under image guidance.
C. The lesion may be malignant and should be surgically biopsied.
D. The lesion is malignant and should be surgically resected with a wide margin.

23 A patient presents with a history of painless swelling along the volar margin of the wrist. What is the most likely diagnosis?

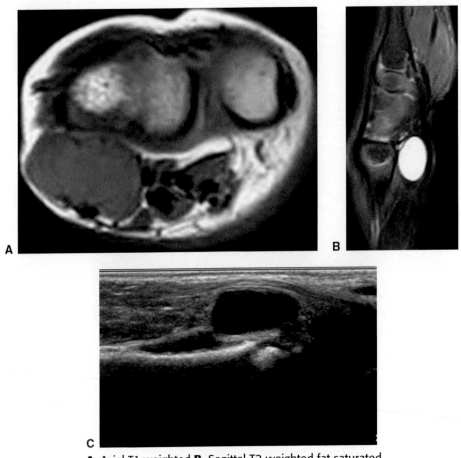

A. Axial T1 weighted **B.** Sagittal T2 weighted fat saturated
C. Ultrasound long axis

   A. Ganglion
   B. Giant cell tumor of tendon sheath
   C. Synovial sarcoma
   D. Nodular synovitis

24 Which of the following lesions most commonly occurs in the epiphysis of a long bone?

   A. Unicameral bone cyst
   B. Enchondroma
   C. Chondroblastoma
   D. Osteochondroma

25 Lymphangiomas are benign, primarily soft tissue tumors composed of lymphoid tissue lined by lymphatic endothelium. Where are they most commonly located?

   A. Axilla
   B. Abdomen
   C. Neck
   D. Lower extremities

26 A 77-year-old male complains of right hip pain 2 years following total hip replacement arthroplasty. What is the most likely diagnosis?

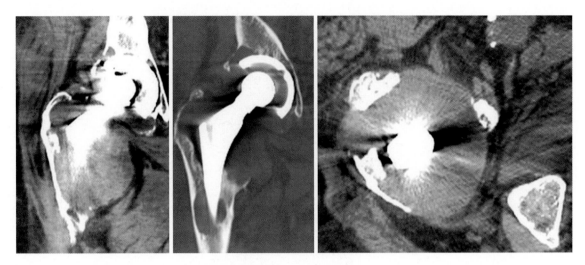

    A. Multiple myeloma
    B. Lytic form of Paget disease
    C. Chondrosarcoma
    D. Periprosthetic osteolysis

27a What type of matrix is present in the humeral lesion depicted in the radiograph?

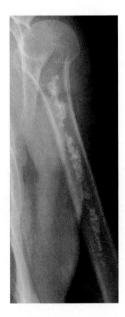

    A. Chondroid
    B. Fibrous
    C. Lipoid
    D. Osseous

27b Which of the following radiologic features best differentiates enchondroma from chondrosarcoma?

    A. Endosteal scalloping
    B. Chondroid matrix
    C. Pathologic fracture
    D. Soft tissue mass

28a A 19-year-old female presents with pain and the following radiographs. What is the most likely diagnosis of the lesion in the proximal phalanx?

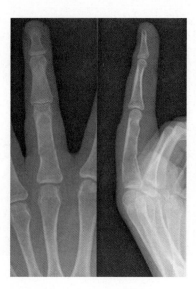

A. Nonossifying fibroma
B. Chondrosarcoma
C. Osteochondroma
D. Enchondroma

28b What is the best management option for this lesion?

A. Radiographic follow-up in 6 months
B. Chemotherapy
C. Surgical curettage and bone grafting
D. Digit amputation

29 A 42-year-old male presents with the following radiograph. Pathologic analysis described the lesion as a mixture of histologic elements. What is the most likely diagnosis?

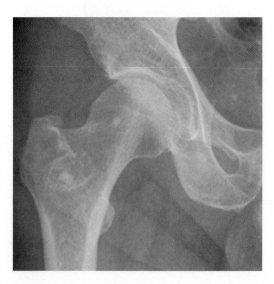

A. Lymphangioma
B. Hemangiopericytoma
C. Liposclerosing myxofibrous tumor
D. Langerhans cell histiocytosis

30a A 30-year-old female presents with the following radiograph and T1-weighted MR image of her ankle. What is the predominant composition of this lesion?

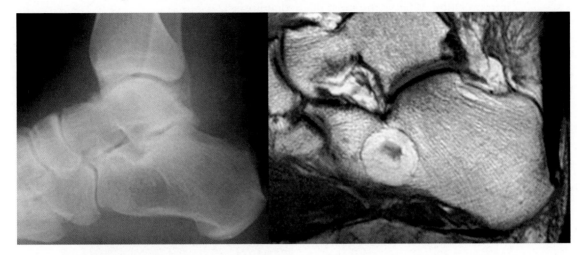

    A. Fat
    B. Neural
    C. Cystic
    D. Fibrous

30b The histologic grade of the lesion would be best described as which of the following?

    A. Benign
    B. Locally aggressive
    C. Low-grade malignant
    D. High-grade malignant

31a Which of the following is a typical MR imaging feature of an intraosseous hemangioma?

    A. Coarsened trabeculae
    B. Diffusely low signal intensity on T1-weighted images
    C. Diffusely low signal intensity on T2-weighted images
    D. No enhancement following contrast administration

31b Where are intraosseous hemangiomas most commonly located?

    A. Femur
    B. Rib
    C. Vertebral body
    D. Calcaneus

32a Sarcomatous degeneration occurs in approximately what percentage of patients with Paget disease with limited skeletal involvement?

    A. 1%
    B. 10% to 15%
    C. 25% to 30%
    D. 50%

32b What is the most common sarcoma associated with Paget degeneration?

    A. Chondrosarcoma
    B. Fibrosarcoma
    C. Osteosarcoma
    D. Malignant fibrous histiocytoma of the bone

33a A 61-year-old male presents with a 2-year history of right shoulder pain. You are presented a radiograph and sagittal T2-weighted fat saturated MR image for interpretation. What is the most likely diagnosis?

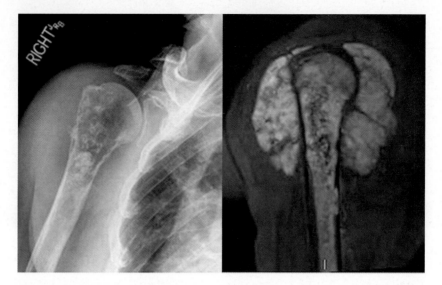

A. Osteosarcoma
B. Chondrosarcoma
C. Malignant fibrous histiocytoma (undifferentiated pleomorphic sarcoma)
D. Giant cell tumor

33b Where is the most common site of metastasis from primary chondrosarcoma?

A. Liver
B. Brain
C. Lung
D. Lymph nodes

33c Which of the following is the most common site of origin for primary chondrosarcoma?

A. Innominate bone
B. Ribs
C. Tibia
D. Spine

34 This 70-year-old male presented with an osseous and soft tissue mass in his left pelvis. He has a history of external beam pelvic radiation for prostate cancer. Osteosarcoma was diagnosed from the percutaneous biopsy. Which of the following dose options is most commonly associated with radiation-induced sarcoma?

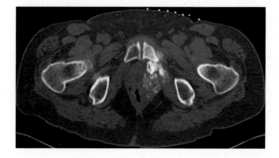

A. 100 cGy
B. 5,500 cGy
C. 7,500 cGy
D. 10,000 cGy

35   A 15-year-old female presents with left thigh pain. Based on the following radiograph and MR images, what is the most likely diagnosis?

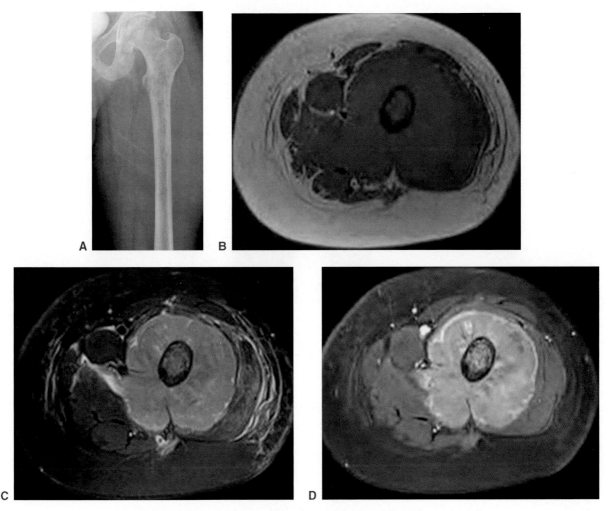

A. Radiograph **B.** Axial T1 weighted **C.** Axial T2 weighted fat saturated
D. Axial T1 weighted fat saturated postcontrast

A. Chondrosarcoma
B. Ewing sarcoma
C. Parosteal osteosarcoma
D. Periosteal osteosarcoma

36a   In Langerhans cell histiocytosis, osseous lesions are the most common disease manifestation. Which of the following is the most common location of extraosseous disease involvement?

A. Lungs
B. Skin
C. Lymph nodes
D. Salivary glands

36b   Which of the following is the most common mean age range at diagnosis?

A. 0 to 10
B. 10 to 20
C. 20 to 30
D. 30 to 40

37a A 29-year-old male presents with the following images of his left forearm. What type of matrix is present in the osseous lesion in the proximal radius?

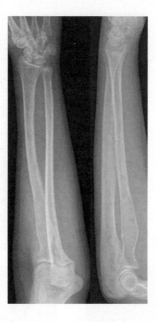

A. Chondroid
B. Fibrous
C. Lipoid
D. Osseous

37b McCune-Albright syndrome is defined as polyostotic fibrous dysplasia in conjunction with

A. pulmonary hypertension.
B. cardiomegaly.
C. endocrine abnormalities.
D. renal agenesis.

38 A 70-year-old patient presents to an orthopedic oncologist with the diagnosis of a bone tumor. Based on the following image, what is the diagnosis?

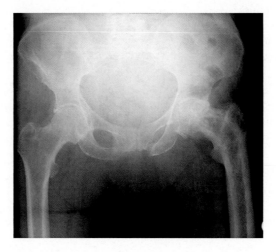

A. Osteosarcoma
B. Paget disease
C. Sclerotic bone metastases
D. Fibrous dysplasia

39a Myxomas are characterized pathologically as lesions with abundant myxoid stroma and bland spindle cells. These features result in which of the following MR imaging appearance?

A. Hyperintensity on T1 weighted
B. Hyperintensity on T2 weighted
C. Blooming on T2* gradient echo
D. No internal enhancement

39b Myxomas have a predication for which of the following tissues?

A. Bone
B. Fascia
C. Muscle
D. Fat

39c Mazabraud syndrome is characterized by myxomas and which of the following?

A. Fibrous dysplasia
B. Enchondromas
C. Neurofibromas
D. Soft tissue hemangiomas

40 An otherwise healthy patient presented with nonspecific shoulder complaints. This radiograph was obtained at the time of initial evaluation. A diagnosis of Gorham disease (Gorham-Stout syndrome) was entertained. Which of the following would best support the proposed diagnosis?

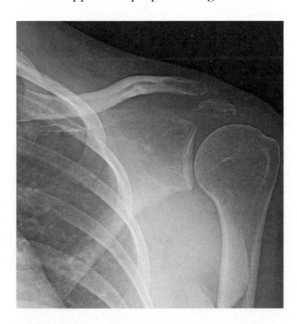

A. History of prior trauma
B. Pathologic fracture
C. Widespread destructive lesions
D. Splenic lesions

41a What would be the most accurate radiographic description of the metadiaphyseal tibial lesion?

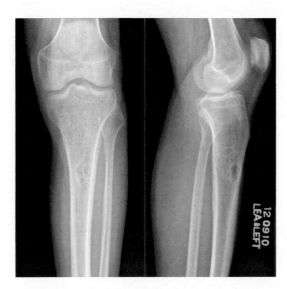

   A. Septated, eccentric, geographic lucent lesion with no identifiable matrix
   B. Expansile, bubbly lytic lesion with chondroid matrix
   C. Well-defined, elongated lytic lesion with osseous matrix
   D. Expansile, eccentric, geographic lucent lesion with osseous matrix

41b Which of the following would be the most likely diagnosis?
   A. Aneurysmal bone cyst
   B. Chondroblastoma
   C. Chondromyxoid fibroma
   D. Metastasis
   E. Osteoblastoma

42 A 70-year-old man presents to his primary physician with the following radiograph and bone scan. Based on the images, what is the most likely diagnosis of the lesion in the left ilium adjacent to the sacroiliac joint?

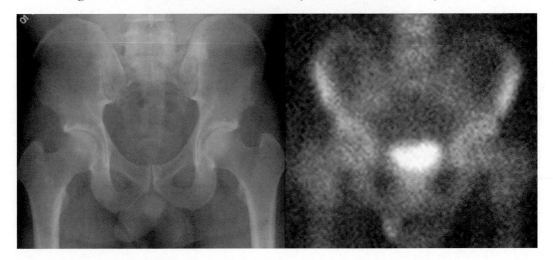

   A. Untreated, sclerotic bone metastasis
   B. Giant bone island
   C. Osteoblastoma
   D. Multiple myeloma

43 Given the imaging findings, which of the following choices should be included in the differential diagnosis?

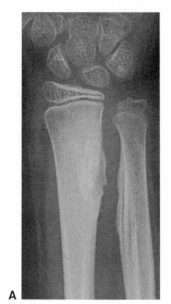
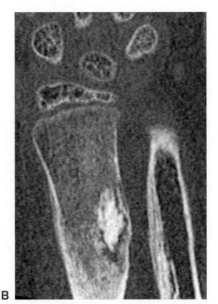
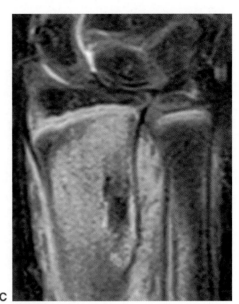

A.

B.

C.

A. Radiograph **B.** Coronal CT **C.** Coronal proton density fat saturated

- A. Osteoid osteoma
- B. Chondroblastoma
- C. Chondrosarcoma
- D. Osteoblastoma
- E. Metastasis

44a A patient with distal thumb tenderness undergoes MRI of the hand with axial T1-weighted, axial T1-weighted fat-saturated postcontrast, and coronal MR angiography images provided. Based on the imaging findings, what is the most likely diagnosis?

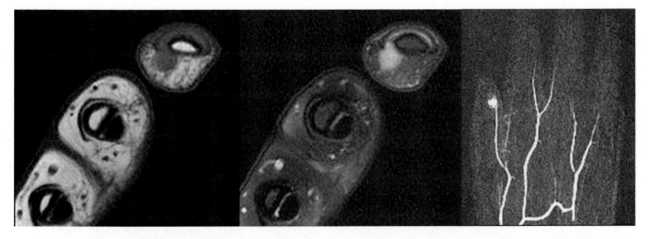

- A. Melanoma
- B. Glomus tumor
- C. Giant cell tumor of the tendon sheath
- D. Mucoid cyst
- E. Epithelial inclusion cyst

44b What is the most common treatment of this lesion?

    A. Embolization
    B. Methotrexate
    C. Radiation
    D. Surgical excision

45 The multiple osseous lesions demonstrated in these radiographs best match with which of the following possibilities?

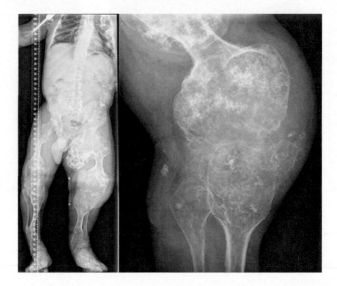

    A. Multiple osteochondromas in the setting of multiple hereditary exostoses
    B. Multiple nonossifying fibromas in the setting of Jaffe-Campanacci syndrome
    C. Multiple enchondromas in the setting of Maffucci syndrome
    D. Multiple osteochondromas and enchondromas in the setting of metachondromatosis
    E. Multiple nonossifying fibromas in the setting of neurofibromatosis type 1

46 Lateral radiograph and axial and sagittal T1-weighted fat-saturated postcontrast images of the thumb are shown. The MRI demonstrates an avidly enhancing soft tissue mass with underlying bony erosions. Which of the following possible differential considerations is the most likely diagnosis given the radiographic and MRI findings?

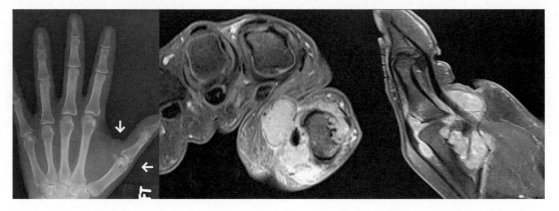

    A. Ganglion cyst
    B. Giant cell tumor of the tendon sheath
    C. Hemangioma
    D. Infection

• **47** AP standing radiograph, axial CT, and axial T2-weighted fat saturated MR images demonstrate a densely mineralized mass in a 64-year-old man. Based on the imaging findings, what is the most likely diagnosis?

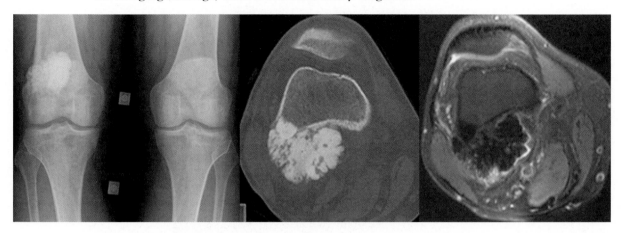

    A. Osteochondroma
    B. Myositis ossificans
    C. Parosteal osteosarcoma
    D. Periosteal chondroma
    E. Periosteal osteosarcoma

48 Differentiation between aneurysmal bone cyst and telangiectatic osteosarcoma on MRI can be difficult given both of these lesions demonstrate fluid-filled hemorrhagic spaces with characteristic fluid–fluid levels. In the case presented, which of the following imaging features suggests the correct diagnosis of telangiectatic osteosarcoma?

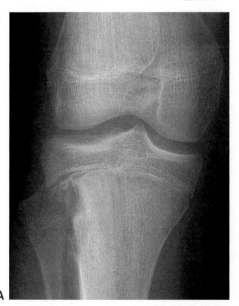
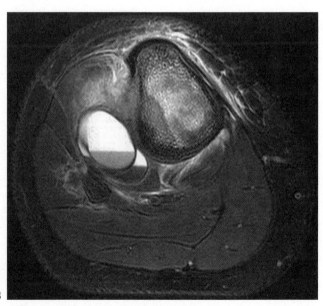

A   B

A. Radiograph **B.** Axial T2 weighted fat saturated

    A. Thick nodular septations on MRI
    B. Cortical destruction
    C. Expansile remodeling
    D. Eccentric location of lesion

49 In this patient presenting with nonspecific fullness along the anterior aspect of the ankle, the addition of what MR imaging sequence would be most helpful in confirming a suspected diagnosis of pigmented villonodular synovitis?

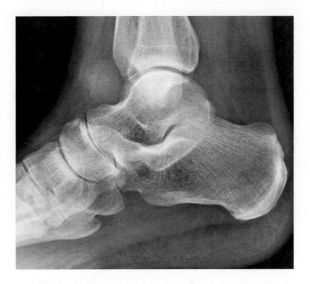

A. Proton density
B. T1 weighted, fat saturated
C. T2* gradient echo
D. Contrast enhanced T1 weighted, fat saturated

50 Pronounced bone marrow edema surrounding the lesion shown in the radiograph would be most characteristic of which of the following?

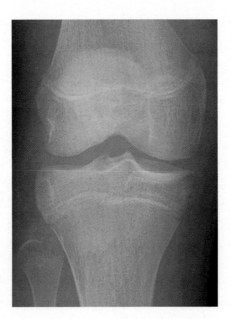

A. Chondroblastoma
B. Giant cell tumor
C. Enchondroma
D. Fibroxanthoma

51 This patient presented with a destructive lesion involving the right scapula. An MRI was obtained for further characterization. Based on the images presented, which of the following would be considered the most likely diagnosis?

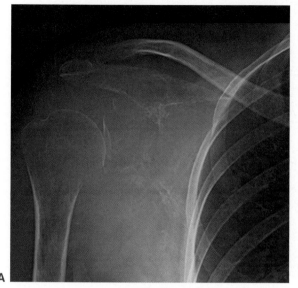 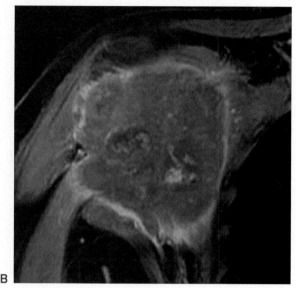

A. Radiograph **B.** Coronal T1 weighted fat saturated postcontrast

    A. Angiosarcoma
    B. Hemangioma
    C. Plasmacytoma
    D. Lymphoma

52 Regarding the images below, which of the following is the best diagnosis?

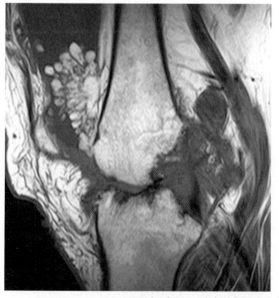 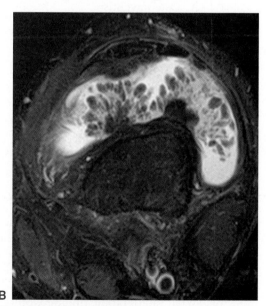

A. Sgittal T1 weighted **B.** Axial T2 weighted fat saturated

    A. Pigmented villonodular synovitis (PVNS)
    B. Synovial chondromatosis
    C. Lipoma arborescens
    D. Synovial hemangioma

53a Which of the following best characterizes the pattern of periosteal reaction demonstrated on the radiographs?

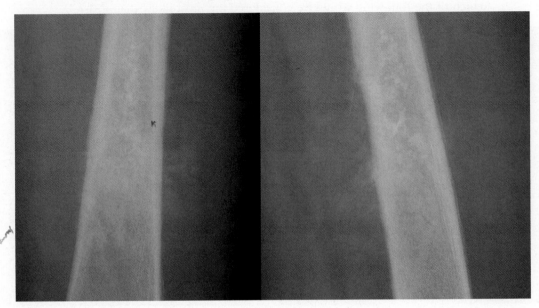

A. Septated
B. Laminated (onion skin)
C. Disorganized
D. Spiculated (sunburst)

53b This pattern of periosteal reaction is most commonly associated with which of the following?

A. Osteomyelitis
B. Eosinophilic granuloma
C. Conventional osteosarcoma
D. Chondroblastoma

54 Which of the following malignancies has the best long-term prognosis?

A. Periosteal osteosarcoma
B. High grade surface osteosarcoma
C. Parosteal osteosarcoma
D. Conventional osteosarcoma
E. Telangiectatic osteosarcoma

55 Which of the following has the highest prevalence of malignant transformation?

A. Enchondroma in Ollier disease or Maffucci syndrome
B. Osteochondroma in multiple hereditary exostoses
C. Nonossifying fibromas in Jaffe-Campanacci syndrome
D. Osteoma in Gardner syndrome

56 What radiographic finding would be diagnostic of a hemangioma in the hand?

A. Bony erosion
B. Soft tissue mass
C. Phleboliths
D. Cortical thickening

57 With regard to conventional osteosarcoma (high-grade intramedullary osteosarcoma), what percentage of cases have pulmonary metastases at the time of diagnosis?

A. 0% to 5%
B. 5% to 10%
C. 10% to 15%
D. 15% to 20%

58 Which of the following statements regarding the radiographic appearance of malignant fibrous histiocytoma (MFH) of the bone is most accurate?

A. Lacks periosteal reaction
B. Lacks a soft tissue mass
C. Presence of cortical expansion
D. Presence of a sclerotic margin

59a Regarding nodular fasciitis, where do lesions most frequently occur?

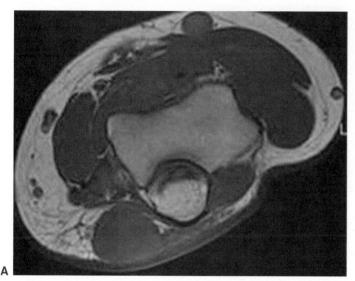 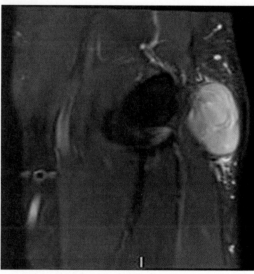

A

B

A. Axial T1 weighted **B.** Sagittal T2 weighted fat saturated

A. Trunk
B. Head and neck
C. Upper extremities
D. Lower extremities

59b The diagnosis of nodular fasciitis was made from a percutaneous biopsy. Of the following, which is the best treatment option?

A. Marginal surgical excision
B. Radical surgical excision
C. Chemotherapy
D. Radiation therapy

60 Regarding adamantinomas, which of the following is a characteristic imaging feature?

A. Expansile
B. Homogeneously sclerotic
C. Wide zone of transition
D. Sunburst periosteal reaction

61a A 60-year-old female presents with asymmetric enlargement of her left thigh. An MRI was performed. Based on the provided images, what is the most likely diagnosis?

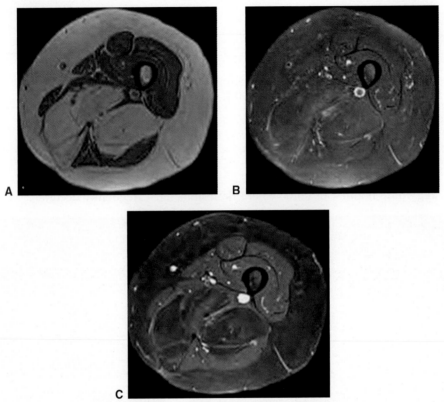

A. Axial T1 weighted B. Axial T2 weighted fat saturated
C. Axial T1 weighted fat saturated postcontrast

A. Well-differentiated liposarcoma (atypical lipomatous tumor)
B. Myxoid liposarcoma
C. Pleomorphic liposarcoma
D. Dedifferentiated liposarcoma

61b The lesion was surgically resected with clear margins. Which radiologic follow-up option is most appropriate?

A. MRI of the thigh to evaluate for local recurrence
B. MRI of the thigh to evaluate for local recurrence and CT chest to evaluate for metastatic disease
C. FDG-PET to evaluate for metastatic disease
D. MRI of the thigh to evaluate for local recurrence and nuclear medicine bone scan to evaluate for metastatic disease

62 A 70-year-old male presents with a soft tissue mass. On MRI, the lesion is a well-defined solid mass with smooth margins and homogeneous signal intensity. The lesion does not contain fat. What is the next best step in this patient's care?

A. No further intervention is necessary as the lesion is benign given the above imaging description.
B. 6-month follow-up is recommended as the lesion is indeterminate.
C. Percutaneous or surgical biopsy is recommended since soft tissue sarcomas may have a bland appearance on MR.
D. Ultrasound to further attempt to characterize fat within the lesion.

· **63** A 25-year-old male presents with anterior knee pain. Two, consecutive
T2-weighted fat-saturated and a T1-weighted fat-saturated postcontrast MR
images are presented for interpretation. What is the most likely diagnosis?

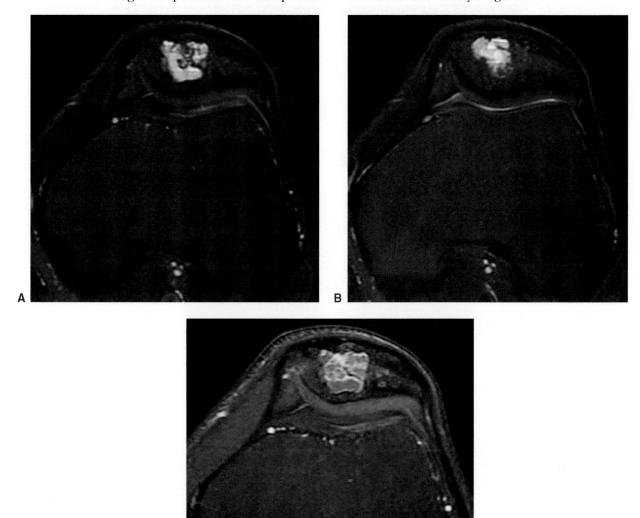

A. Axial T2 weighted fat saturated **B.** Axial T2 weighted fat saturated
C. Axial T1 weighted fat saturated postcontrast

A. Giant cell tumor
B. Aneurysmal bone cyst
C. Osteomyelitis
D. Brown tumor in hyperparathyroidism

· **64** Which of the following most accurately describes the cellular origin of
hemangioendotheliomas?

A. Tumor arising from smooth muscle cells of blood vessels
B. Tumor arising from collagen fibers in the tunica adventitia of blood vessels
C. Tumor of endothelial cells or their precursors
D. Tumor of abnormal proliferation of red blood cells

65 A 60-year-old male presents with the following radiographs. What is the most likely diagnosis?

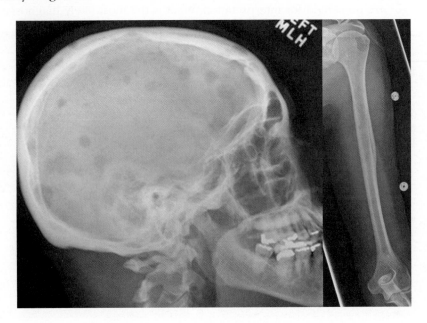

    A. Primary osteoporosis
    B. Lymphangioma
    C. Prostate metastases
    D. Multiple myeloma

66 An 18-year-old female presents with the following radiograph and MR images of her left humerus. What is the most likely diagnosis?

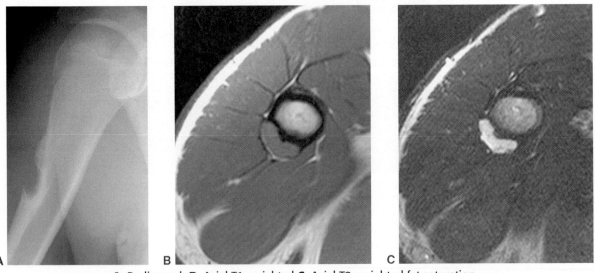

A. Radiograph **B.** Axial T1 weighted **C.** Axial T2 weighted fat saturation

    A. Myositis ossificans
    B. Periosteal desmoid
    C. Osteochondroma
    D. Periosteal chondroma

67 Which of the following paraneoplastic syndromes is associated with hemangiopericytomas (solitary fibrous tumor)?

A. Hypoglycemia
B. Hyperglycemia
C. Hyperphosphatemia
D. Hypercalcemia

68 A 16-year-old male presents with a lesion in his proximal tibia. Which of the following is the recommended biopsy path?

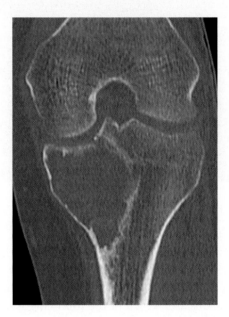

A. Anteromedial
B. Anterolateral
C. Posteromedial
D. Posterolateral

69 Periosteal and parosteal osteosarcomas are surface lesions. Which of the following imaging appearance is more characteristic of a periosteal osteosarcoma?

A. Mature bone extending from the center of the lesion to the periphery.
B. Bone marrow is nearly always involved.
C. "Sunburst" appearance due to calcified spicules of the bone perpendicular to the cortex.
D. Neoplastic cortical thickening rarely with an associated soft tissue mass.

70 A patient presents with a disseminated, hamartomatous disorder composed of hemangiomatous and lymphangiomatous lesions in the axial and appendicular skeletal and visceral organ involvement. Which of the following diagnoses is accurate?

A. Mastocytosis
B. Cystic angiomatosis
C. Langerhans cell histiocytosis
D. Multiple myeloma

71 Which of the following most accurately describes the margin of the lesion in the humerus?

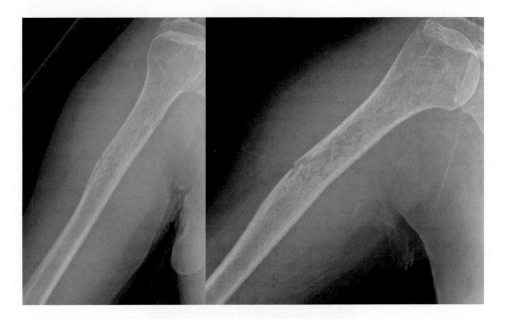

A. Geographic, well defined with no sclerotic margin
B. Nongeographic, well defined with no sclerotic margin
C. Geographic, ill defined
D. Nongeographic, permeative

72 A 70-year-old male presents with right wrist pain and the following radiograph. Assuming metastatic disease, which of the following is the most likely primary tumor?

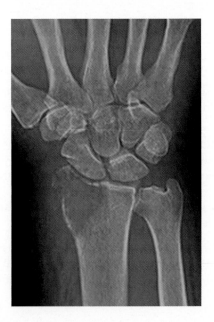

A. Renal cell carcinoma
B. Neuroblastoma
C. Prostate carcinoma
D. Papillary thyroid carcinoma

• **73** Regarding osseous lymphoma, which of the following imaging features is accurate?

    A. Primarily occurs in the epiphysis of long bones

    B. Primarily a sclerotic lesion with a dense tumor matrix.

    C. Periosteal reaction is uncommon.

    D. Often associated with a soft tissue mass.

° **74** A 25-year-old female presents with the history of a neck mass for 2 years. Which of the following is the most likely natural history of the tumor noted in the images below?

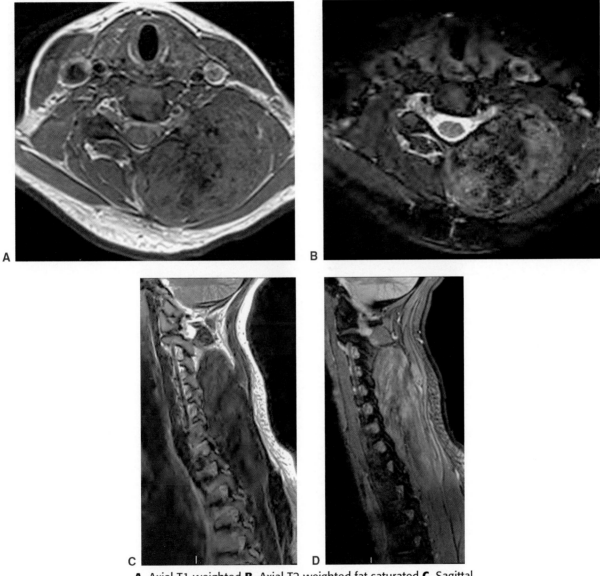

A. Axial T1 weighted **B.** Axial T2 weighted fat saturated **C.** Sagittal T2 weighted fat saturated **D.** Sagittal T2 gradient echo

    A. The lesion has stabilized in size since the patient is skeletally mature.

    B. Regression over time with areas of dystrophic calcification and cyst formation

    C. Invasion of the adjacent neural foramina

    D. Metastatic disease to the lungs and liver

75 A 65-year-old female presents with the following soft tissue mass in her right thigh. Statistically, which of the following options represents the most likely diagnosis?

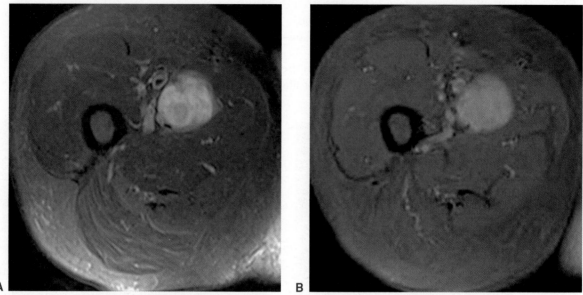

A. Axial T2 weighted fat saturated **B.** Axial T1 weighted fat saturated postcontrast

A. Pleomorphic liposarcoma
B. Leiomyosarcoma
C. Synovial sarcoma
D. Malignant fibrous histiocytoma (undifferentiated pleomorphic sarcoma)

ANSWERS AND EXPLANATIONS

1   **Answer B.**   Ollier disease is a nonhereditary dysplasia characterized by the presence of multiple enchondromas. These lesions commonly involve the metaphyseal regions of the long bones and are characteristically unilateral or asymmetric. The skull and spine are spared. Lesions usually regress or stabilize after skeletal maturation. The enchondromas can result in growth disturbance, bowing deformities, and increased risk of sarcomatous degeneration (due primarily to their multiplicity). MR features of these chondroid lesions include lobular margins and internal hyperintensity on T2-weighted MRI.

Reference: Greenspan A, Gernot J, Remagen W. *Differential Diagnosis in Orthopaedic Oncology.* 2nd ed. Philadelphia, PA: Lippincott Williams & Wilkins; 2007:169–172.

2   **Answer C.**   The majority of cases of Ewing sarcoma are metadiaphyseal in location (44% to 59%), followed by diaphyseal in 33% to 35% and metaphyseal in 5% to 15%. Lesions originating in the epiphysis are rare.

Reference: Murphey MD, Senchak LT, Mambalam PK, et al. From the radiologic pathology archives: Ewing sarcoma family of tumors: radiologic-pathologic correlation. *Radiographics.* 2013;33:803–831.

3   **Answer C.**   Plantar fibromatosis is classified as a type of fibroblastic and myofibroblastic tumor. It accounts for 2.3% of benign tumors of the foot. It is more common in men and bilateral in 20% to 50% of cases. On ultrasound, the lesion is identified as a nodular area in the plantar fascia that is hypoechoic or heterogenous. T1-weighted MRI demonstrates low to isointense signal intensity and fluid sensitive sequences demonstrate heterogeneous signal intensity. Contrast enhancement is variable. Fibromatosis usually occurs at the medial non–weight-bearing surface of the plantar fascia. Forestier disease is also known as diffuse idiopathic skeletal hyperostosis (DISH) and involves the spine. Plantar fasciopathy or fasciitis is the most common cause of heel pain and is characterized by thickening of the fascia, usually at the calcaneal margin, with variable degrees of soft tissue and osseous inflammation. Morton neuroma is mass-like fibrosis of the plantar digital nerve, at the level of the metatarsal heads, most commonly between the second and third intermetatarsal spaces.

References: Berquist T. *Imaging of the Foot and Ankle.* 3rd ed. Philadelphia, PA: Lippincott Williams & Wilkins; 2011:417.

Narvaez JA, Narvaez J, Ortega R, et al. Painful heel: MR imaging findings. *Radiographics.* 2000;20:333–352.

4   **Answer B.**   There are a number of features when found within a fatty, soft tissue lesion that should raise suspicion for a possible malignancy such as a liposarcoma. These features include thick septations measuring >2 mm, lesion size larger than 10 cm, and the presence of globular or nodular nonadipose areas.

References: Gaskin CM, Helms CA. Lipomas, lipoma variants, and well-differentiated liposarcomas (atypical lipomas): results of MRI evaluations of 126 consecutive fatty masses. *AJR Am J Roentgenol.* 2004;182:733–739.

Kransdorf MJ, Bancroft LW, Peterson JJ, et al. Imaging of fatty tumors: distinction of lipoma and well-differentiated liposarcoma. *Radiology.* 2002;224:99–104.

5 **Answer B.** The iliac bone is the most frequent site used for bone graft. It allows for a variety of types of bone, mostly cancellous, and for a variety of uses. The anterior iliac crest is the most easily assessed site for grafting.

Reference: Kai-Uwe L. *Advances in Spinal Fusion: Molecular Science, Biomechanics, and Clinical Management.* Monticello, NY: Marcel Dekker; 2004:687.

6 **Answer B.** Pigmented villonodular synovitis (PVNS) is depicted in the MR images provided. The MR features of PVNS include a synovial based lesion, joint effusion, and osseous erosions, which are more commonly found in the less capacious joints such as the hip, shoulder, elbow, and ankle. In addition, the tendency of these lesions to bleed results in hemosiderin deposition and the associated paramagnetic effects of hemosiderin, which includes a decrease in signal intensity in all pulse sequences, and "blooming" artifact on the gradient-echo sequence. Hemophilic arthropathy, with its repetitive bleeding into the synovial joints, can also lead to absorption of hemosiderin by the synovium and would be a differential consideration.

References: Murphey MD, Rhee JH, Lewis RB, et al. Pigmented villonodular synovitis: radiologic-pathologic correlation. *Radiographics.* 2008;28:1493–1518.

Narváez JA, Narváez J, Ortega R, et al. Hypointense synovial lesions on T2-weighted images: differential diagnosis with pathologic correlation. *AJR Am J Roentgenol.* 2003;181:761–769.

7 **Answer B.** The question describes the classic appearance of a giant cell tumor, which is located in the metaphysis with epiphyseal extension typically to the subarticular margin. The majority of these tumors occur between the ages of 20 and 50, with peak incidence in the third decade of life. Giant cell tumors may also exhibit radiographically aggressive features such as expansile remodeling, cortical thinning or breakthrough, soft tissue mass, and a wide zone of transition.

Reference: Chakarun CJ, Forrester DM, Gottsegen CJ, et al. Giant cell tumor of bone: review, mimics, and new developments in treatment. *Radiographics.* 2013;33:197–211.

8 **Answer A.** Intramuscular hemangiomas are benign tumors with vascular channels. They demonstrate high T2-weighted MR signal, due to slow flow, with enhancement on postcontrast images. Phleboliths may be seen on radiographs, which may be diagnostic.

References: Cohen EK, Kressel HY, Perosio T, et al. MR imaging of soft-tissue masses: correlation with pathologic findings. *AJR Am J Roentgenol.* 1988;150:1079–1081.

Provenzale J, Nelson R. *Duke Radiology Case Review: Imaging, Differential Diagnosis, and Discussion.* Philadelphia, PA: Lippincott-Raven; 1998:269.

9 **Answer A.** Nonossifying fibroma (synonyms: fibroxanthoma, benign fibrous cortical defect) is typically a "do not touch" lesion, but if associated with a pathologic fracture, curettage and bone grafting may be indicated.

Reference: Manaster BJ, Roberts CC, Petersilge CA, et al. *Diagnostic Imaging: Musculoskeletal: Non-Traumatic Disease.* Manitoba, Canada: Amirsys; 2010;2:218–221.

10 **Answer D.** The nuclear bone scan shows heterogeneous, multifocal areas of abnormal osseous uptake throughout the axial and appendicular skeleton, with decreased renal tracer uptake, compatible with a superscan. The correlative radiographic findings show patchy sclerotic lesions within the left femur, with associated ill-defined periosteal reaction. The imaging is consistent with diffuse, osteoblastic metastatic disease.

Reference: Manaster BJ, Roberts CC, Petersilge CA, et al. *Diagnostic Imaging: Musculoskeletal: Non-Traumatic Disease.* Manitoba, Canada: Amirsys; 2010;2:138–143.

11 **Answer B.** Osteofibrous dysplasia is a developmental tumor-like, fibroosseous condition with a tendency toward spontaneous regression and without significant residual skeletal deformity. Osteofibrous dysplasia is found, almost exclusively, within the tibial diaphysis and typically involves the anterior cortex. Osseous bowing, osseous enlargement, and intracortical osteolysis with a characteristic adjacent sclerotic band are typically seen on radiographs. From an imaging standpoint, distinction between osteofibrous dysplasia, adamantinoma, and fibrous dysplasia may be challenging; however, they are better differentiated pathologically.

References: Lee RS, Weitze S, Eastwood DM, et al. Osteofibrous dysplasia of the tibia. Is there a need for a radical surgical approach? *J Bone Joint Surg Br.* 2006;88:658–664.
Levine SM, Lambiase RE, Petchprapa CN. Cortical lesions of the tibia: characteristic appearances at conventional radiography. *Radiographics.* 2003;23:157–177.

12 **Answer D.** This is a biopsy-proven bizarre parosteal osteochondromatous proliferation (BPOP). BPOP, otherwise known as "Nora lesion," was first described by Dr. Frederick E. Nora et al. in 1983. BPOPs are rare, exophytic growths from osseous cortical surfaces consisting of bone, cartilage, and fibrous tissue. Some studies suggest the etiology of this lesion to be related to a reparative process after periosteal injury, while others point to a benign neoplastic process as its cause. Osteochondromas must demonstrate corticomedullary contiguity. Osteosarcoma and Ewing sarcoma are rare in this location and would have a more aggressive appearance. Myositis ossificans is benign, heterotopic ossification occurring within skeletal muscle, usually within large muscles.

References: Dhondt E, Oudenhoven L, Khan S, et al. Nora lesion, a distinct radiological entity? *Skeletal Radiol.* 2006;35:497–502.
Meneses MF, Unni KK, Swee RG. Bizarre parosteal osteochondromatous proliferation of bone (Nora lesion). *Am J Surg Pathol.* 1993;17:691–697.

13 **Answer B.** The image depicts an osseous lesion of the skull, most consistent with an osteoma. Osteomas commonly involve the skull, paranasal sinuses, and mandible. They are typically asymptomatic, though they may result in hearing, vision, and breathing symptoms depending on their size and location. They are typically benign and require no treatment unless they become symptomatic. Osteomas can be seen in association with Gardner syndrome, an intestinal polyposis syndrome. Peutz Jeghers syndrome is also an intestinal polyposis syndrome, but is not associated with osteomas. Maffucci syndrome and Ollier disease are seen in association with multiple enchondromas of the hand.

References: Erdogan N, Demir U, Songu M, et al. A prospective study of paranasal sinus osteomas in 1,889 cases: changing patterns of localization. *Laryngoscope.* 2009;119(12):2355–2359.
Huvos A. *Bone Tumors: Diagnosis, Treatment and Prognosis.* 2nd ed. Philadelphia, PA: Saunders; 1990.
Bullough P. *Orthopaedic Pathology.* 3rd ed. London, England: Times Mirror International Publishers; 1997.

14 **Answer D.** The images demonstrate multiple osseous lesions in a metaphyseal location, consistent with multiple osteochondromas. This entity is known as hereditary multiple exostoses (HME), which is inherited via an autosomal dominant pattern. Patients with HME have an increased risk of a lesion undergoing malignant degeneration to chondrosarcoma when compared to patients with solitary osteochondromas. Approximately 1% to 3% of patients suffer malignant degeneration.

References: Murphey MD, Choi JJ, Kransdorf MJ, et al. Imaging of osteochondroma: variants and complications with radiologic-pathologic correlation. *Radiographics.* 2000;20:1407–1434.
Peterson HA. Multiple hereditary osteochondromata. *Clin Orthop.* 1989;239:222–230.

15 Answer D. When the parent nerve is identified, an eccentrically positioned lesion in relation to the nerve suggests a schwannoma. The target sign seen with peripheral nerve sheath tumors shows increased signal peripherally and more intermediate signal centrally within the lesion on T2-weighted sequences.

The split fat sign is indicated by a thin rim of fat surrounding the lesion, and can be seen with either a neurofibroma or a schwannoma. The fascicular sign demonstrates multiple small ring-like structures, and can also be seen with either a neurofibroma or a schwannoma.

References: Jee WH, Oh SN, McCauley T, et al. Extraaxial neurofibromas versus neurilemmomas: discrimination with MRI. *AJR Am J Roentgenol.* 2004;183(3):629–633.
Lin J, Martel W. Cross-sectional imaging of peripheral nerve sheath tumors characteristic signs on CT, MR imaging, and sonography. *AJR Am J Roentgenol.* 2001;176:75–82.

16 Answer D. There are multiple factors that may suggest a worrisome appearance for malignant transformation of an osteochondroma to a chondrosarcoma. Growth or increased size, in a skeletally mature patient, of a previously unchanged osteochondroma can be an important indicator of malignant transformation. Focal thickening of the cartilage cap of an osteochondroma to >1.5 cm may suggest malignant transformation. Development of focal destruction with lucent foci within the interior of a lesion is a worrisome sign for malignant transformation of an osteochondroma. Development of an irregular or indistinct surface of the lesion is yet another sign of malignant transformation. Development of a fluid signal intensity bursa overlying an osteochondroma, however, is often related to frictional forces between the lesion and the surrounding soft tissues and is not typically associated with malignant transformation.

References: Bernard SA, Murphey MD, Flemming DJ, et al. Improved differentiation of benign osteochondromas from secondary chondrosarcomas with standardized measurement of cartilage cap at CT and MR imaging. *Radiology.* 2010;255:3:857–865.
Murphey MD, Choi JJ, Kransdorf MJ, et al. Imaging of osteochondroma: variants and complications with radiologic-pathologic correlation. *Radiographics.* 2000;20:1407–1434.

17 Answer C. Synovial chondromatosis is a benign disorder characterized by formation of multiple intra-articular nodules composed of hyaline cartilage. It most commonly involves the knee joint, >50% of cases, followed by the elbow, hip and shoulder. 80% of cases have erosions of the adjacent bone, as is seen in the radius in this case. The synovial chondromatosis bodies are most commonly low to intermediate on T1-weighted and hyperintense on T2-weighted MR images. The provided axial and coronal T2-weighted MR images show hyperintense chondromatosis bodies. The synovium typically enhances on contrast-enhanced images. Low signal and blooming artifact are most commonly associated with pigmented villonodular synovitis. Malignant transformation from synovial chondromatosis to chondrosarcoma has been described but is rare.

References: Buddingh EP, Krallman P, Neff JR, et al. Chromosome 6 abnormalities are recurrent in synovial chondromatosis. *Cancer Genet Cytogenet.* 2003;140:18–22.
Murphey MD, Vidal JA, Fanburg-Smith JC, et al. Imaging of synovial chondromatosis with radiologic-pathologic correlation. *Radiographics.* 2007;27:1465–1488.

18 Answer A. The image depicts an osteoid osteoma. The most common location is the cortex of long bones. The most common long bone is the femur followed by the tibia; collectively, these account for 60% of cases. Intramedullary location is rare. For intracapsular lesions, the most common location is the femoral neck. In the spine, the most common location is the lumbar spine (59%), followed by the cervical spine, thoracic spine, and sacrum. Patients frequently present with pain that is local and worse at night, which is typically relieved by nonsteroidal anti-inflammatory medications. It occurs in young patients between the ages of 5 and 40 years of age. Image-guided radiofrequency ablation or other forms of thermal ablation are the preferred treatment for osteoid osteoma. Surgical resection is also an option; however, only the lucent nidus needs to be resected. The surrounding sclerosis and periosteal reaction is reactive and does not need to be resected for successful treatment.

References: Gangi A, Alizadeh H, Wong L, et al. Osteoid osteoma: percutaneous laser ablation and follow-up in 114 patients. *Radiology.* 2007;242:293–301.
Manaster BJ, Roberts CC, Petersilge CA, et al. *Diagnostic Imaging: Musculoskeletal: Non-Traumatic Disease.* Manitoba, Canada: Amirsys; 2010;2:26–31.

19 Answer C.   Coronal T1-weighted and axial T2-weighted MR images are presented in this case. Synovial sarcoma histologically resembles synovial tissue but does not necessarily arise from synovial tissue. These sarcomas typically occur near a joint or within a tendon sheath, but less commonly occurs within the joint itself. It is most commonly seen in the lower extremity, particularly the popliteal fossa about the knee. However, synovial sarcomas can involve nearly any site in the body. Synovial sarcoma can be seen in any age group but is most commonly seen in young adults. Males are affected slightly more commonly than females. Synovial sarcoma will demonstrate internal mineralization on radiographs in nearly one-third of all cases. On MRI, this mineralization presents as areas of low signal intensity. The T1 appearance of synovial sarcoma is most commonly similar to or lower than skeletal muscle. The T2 appearance is typically hyperintense to skeletal muscle. After contrast administration, the tumor demonstrates prominent, heterogeneous enhancement.

References: Murphey MD, Gibson MS, Jennings BT, et al. Imaging of synovial sarcoma with radiologic-pathologic correlation. *Radiographics.* 2006;26:1543–1565.
Nakanishi H, Araki N, Sawai Y, et al. Cystic synovial sarcomas: imaging features with clinical and histopathologic correlation. *Skeletal Radiol.* 2003;32:701–707.

20 Answer A.   The image depicts a simple bone cyst. These are typically centrally located, intramedullary, geographic lytic lesions, often associated with endosteal scalloping and expansile remodeling. They are most commonly metaphyseal, but can occasionally involve the metadiaphysis related to new bone formation between the lesion and the adjacent physis. They are most commonly seen in the proximal humerus, proximal femur, and proximal tibia in the pediatric population. Pathologic fracture through the lesion is commonly seen, with >50% of patients presenting with a pathologic fracture. This fracture may present as a fallen fragment sign with a small fracture fragment migrating through the fluid-filled cyst to the dependent portion of the lesion.

References: Lokiec F, Wientroub S. Simple bone cyst: etiology, classification, pathology, and treatment modalities. *J Pediatr Orthop B.* 1998;7(4):262–273.
Struhl S, Edelson C, Pritzker H, et al. Solitary (unicameral) bone cyst. The fallen fragment sign revisited. *Skeletal Radiol.* 1989;18(4):261–265.

21 Answer A.   Approach A traverses the deltoid musculature anteriorly just lateral to the deltopectoral interval, which is typically the ideal approach for proximal humeral biopsies. The deltoid is innervated from posterior to anterior, and therefore, biopsies and surgical incisions are typically performed via an anterior approach. Approach B utilizes an anterolateral approach that is suboptimal compared to approach A. Approaches C and D use a posterolateral and posterior approach that should be avoided.

References: Anderson MW, Temple HT, Dussault RG, et al. Compartmental anatomy: relevance to staging and biopsy of musculoskeletal tumors. *AJR Am J Roentgenol* 1999;173:1663–1671.
Liu PT, Valadez SD, Chivers FS, et al. Anatomically based guidelines for core needle biopsy of bone tumors: implications for limb-sparing surgery. *Radiographics.* 2007;27:189–205.

22 **Answer A.**   The images depict a nonosseous fibroma involving the distal femoral metadiaphysis. The imaging features are characteristic of this lesion, and no further workup is necessary. Therefore, an image-guided or surgical biopsy or a wide excision surgical resection is not required.

References: Moser RP Jr, Sweet DE, Haseman DB. Multiple skeletal fibroxanthomas: radiologic-pathologic correlation of 72 cases. *Skeletal Radiol*. 1987;16(5):353–359.
Smith SE, Kransdorf MJ. Primary musculoskeletal neoplasms of fibrous origin. *Semin Musculoskel Radiol*. 2000;4(1):73–88.

23 **Answer A.**   Ganglion is a benign cystic lesion. The majority of ganglia are located around the wrist. Occasionally, they are seen around other major joints, such as the knee. This lesion is hypointense on T1-weighted and hyperintense on T2-weighted MR images and is cystic on ultrasound. Giant cell tumor of the tendon sheath, nodular synovitis, and synovial sarcoma are solid masses.

Reference: Beaman FD, Peterson JJ. MR imaging of cysts, ganglia, and bursae about the knee. *Radiol Clin North Am*. 2007;45(6):969–982.

24 **Answer C.**   Chondroblastomas most commonly occur in the epiphysis or epiphyseal equivalents of bone and growth may extend into the metaphysis. Unicameral bone cyst, enchondroma, and osteochondromas are benign osseous lesions, which most commonly occur in the metaphysis of the bone.

Reference: Manaster BJ, Roberts CC, Petersilge CA, et al. *Diagnostic Imaging: Musculoskeletal: Non-Traumatic Disease*. Manitoba, Canada: Amirsys; 2010;2:86–87.

25 **Answer C.**   Lymphangiomas are most commonly located in the head and neck, 75%. Approximately 20% are located in the axilla. 50% to 65% of cases are present at birth with 90% of cases are discovered by 2 years of age. Histologic subclassification occurs by vessel composition including capillary, cavernous, cystic, and mixed.

References: Kransdorf MJ, Murphey MD. *Imaging of Soft Tissue Tumors*. 2nd ed. Philadelphia, PA: Lippincott Williams & Wilkins; 2006:165–169.
Murphey MD, Fairbairn KJ, Parman LM, et al. From the archives of the AFIP: musculoskeletal angiomatous lesions: radiologic-pathologic correlation. *Radiographics*. 1995;15:893–917.

26 **Answer D.**   Osteolysis of the pelvis is a common complication following total hip replacement arthroplasty. It is associated with well-defined lucencies surrounding the implant with a narrow zone of transition and endosteal scalloping. Multiple myeloma is usually associated with multiple small, variable-sized lytic lesions and bone demineralization. The majority of chondrosarcomas contain mineralized chondroid matrix. The lytic form of Paget disease is an early phase characterized by osteolysis. In the skull, there are typically large areas of osteolysis most commonly affecting the frontal and occipital bones. In long bones, there is often a sharp demarcation between the advancing osteolytic margin and normal bone, the so-called blade of grass sign.

Reference: Chiang PP, Burke DW, Freiberg AA, et al. Osteolysis of the pelvis: evaluation and treatment. *Clin Orthop Relat Res*. 2003;417:164–174.

27a **Answer A.**   The lesion that spans the proximal humeral metadiaphysis and diaphysis is chondroid composition. Chondroid matrix descriptors include rings and arcs, popcorn, focal stippled, and flocculent. Osseous and fibrous are two other types of bone tumor matrix.

References: Ferrer-Santacreu EM, Ortiz-Cruz EJ, Gonzalez-Lopez JM, et al. Enchondroma versus low-grade chondrosarcoma in appendicular skeleton: clinical and radiological criteria. *J Oncol*. 2012;2012:437958.
Murphey MD, Flemming DJ, Boyea SR, et al. Enchondroma versus chondrosarcoma in the appendicular skeleton: differentiating features. *Radiographics*. 1998;18:1213–1237.

27b **Answer D.** Chondroid matrix, endosteal scalloping, and pathologic fracture may be seen with both enchondromas and chondrosarcomas. Cortical destruction and soft tissue mass are features of chondrosarcoma. Lesional pain and increased uptake on nuclear medicine bone scan (greater than the anterior iliac crest) are also highly suspicious for chondrosarcoma.

References: Ferrer-Santacreu EM, Ortiz-Cruz EJ, Gonzalez-Lopez JM, et al. Enchondroma versus low-grade chondrosarcoma in appendicular skeleton: clinical and radiological criteria. *J Oncol.* 2012;2012:437958.
Murphey MD, Flemming DJ, Boyea SR, et al. Enchondroma versus chondrosarcoma in the appendicular skeleton: differentiating features. *Radiographics.* 1998;18:1213–1237.

28a **Answer D.** The lytic lesion depicted in the proximal phalanx is an enchondroma with a pathologic fracture. Management options include observation versus surgical curettage and grafting.

Reference: Manaster BJ, Roberts CC, Petersilge CA, et al. *Diagnostic Imaging: Musculoskeletal: Non-Traumatic Disease.* Manitoba, Canada: Amirsys; 2010;2:68–73.

28b **Answer C.** In this case, the patient is symptomatic and the lesion has fractured; thus C, surgical curettage and bone grafting, is the best management option. Chemotherapy and amputation are incorrect options as this lesion is benign.

Reference: Manaster BJ, Roberts CC, Petersilge CA, et al. *Diagnostic Imaging: Musculoskeletal: Non-Traumatic Disease.* Manitoba, Canada: Amirsys; 2010;2:68–73.

29 **Answer C.** Liposclerosing myxofibrous tumor is a benign fibro-osseous lesion comprised of a mixture of histologic elements, which may include lipoma, myxoma, myxofibroma, fibroxanthoma, fibrous dysplasia–like features, cyst formation, ischemic ossification, and cartilage. It has a predilection for the intertrochanteric region of the femur. Lesions are often discovered incidentally, but may be related to nonspecific pain or, less commonly, pathologic fracture. Differential considerations include fibrous dysplasia and involuting, intraosseous lipoma. Lymphangioma is a developmental, soft tissue lesion of dilated lymphatic channels. Hemangiopericytoma is a vascular lesion of intermediate malignancy. Langerhans cell histiocytosis is a neoplastic disease primarily of childhood characterized by proliferation of Langerhans cells. Osseous lesions are lytic with radiologic features such as periosteal reaction, endosteal scalloping, cortical breakthrough, and no sclerotic margin.

References: Manaster BJ, Roberts CC, Petersilge CA, et al. *Diagnostic Imaging: Musculoskeletal: Non-Traumatic Disease.* Manitoba, Canada: Amirsys; 2010;2:146–147.
Murphey MD, Carroll JF, Flemming DJ, et al. From the archives of the AFIP: Benign musculoskeletal lipomatous lesions. *Radiographics.* 2004;24:1433–1466.

30a **Answer A.** The calcaneal lesion is an intraosseous lipoma, composed primarily of fat. These lesions are often incidental findings, but may be associated with pain. Pathologic fractures are possible but rare. They are most prevalent in the proximal femur but may also occur in other long bones, calcaneus, ilium, and ribs. Lesions are located in the metaphysis more commonly than the diaphysis, with epiphyseal involvement uncommon. Central or ring-like calcification/ossification in a lucent calcaneal lesion is pathognomonic.

Reference: Murphey MD, Carroll JF, Flemming DJ, et al. From the archives of the AFIP: benign musculoskeletal lipomatous lesions. *Radiographics.* 2004;24:1433–1466.

30b **Answer A.** Intraosseous lipomas are benign lesions and treatment is usually not indicated.

Reference: Murphey MD, Carroll JF, Flemming DJ, et al. From the archives of the AFIP: benign musculoskeletal lipomatous lesions. *Radiographics.* 2004;24:1433–1466.

31a **Answer A.** Intraosseous hemangiomas are characterized by coarsened trabeculations and high signal intensity on T1- and T2-weighted (non–fat-saturated) MR imaging owing to their composition of fat tissue and vascular channels. They characteristically enhance.

Reference: Manaster BJ, Roberts CC, Petersilge CA, et al. *Diagnostic Imaging: Musculoskeletal: Non-Traumatic Disease*. Manitoba, Canada: Amirsys; 2010;2:168–170.

31b **Answer C.** Intraosseous hemangiomas are most commonly located in the vertebral bodies. They may extend to involve the posterior elements or uncommonly involve the posterior elements without vertebral body involvement. Other less common sites of involvement include the calvarium and long bones, specifically the femur, tibia, and humerus.

Reference: Manaster BJ, Roberts CC, Petersilge CA, et al. *Diagnostic Imaging: Musculoskeletal: Non-Traumatic Disease*. Manitoba, Canada: Amirsys; 2010;2:168–170.

32a **Answer A.** The risk of sarcomatous degeneration of pagetoid bone is approximately 1% in individuals with limited skeletal involvement. Sarcomatous degeneration is characterized by cortical destruction with a soft tissue mass.

References: Manaster BJ, Roberts CC, Petersilge CA, et al. *Diagnostic Imaging: Musculoskeletal: Non-Traumatic Disease*. Manitoba, Canada: Amirsys; 2010;2:184–186.
Smith SE, Murphey MD, Motamedi K, et al. From the archives of the AFIP. Radiologic spectrum of Paget disease of bone and its complications with pathologic correlation. *Radiographics*. 2002;22:1191–1216.

32b **Answer C.** Osteosarcoma is the most common lesion associated with degeneration, accounting for 50% to 60% of cases. Malignant fibrous histiocytoma/fibrosarcoma (20% to 25%) and chondrosarcoma (10%) are the next most common lesions.

References: Manaster BJ, Roberts CC, Petersilge CA, et al. *Diagnostic Imaging: Musculoskeletal: Non-Traumatic Disease*. Manitoba, Canada: Amirsys; 2010;2:184–186.
Smith SE, Murphey MD, Motamedi K, et al. From the archives of the AFIP. Radiologic spectrum of Paget disease of bone and its complications with pathologic correlation. *Radiographics*. 2002;22:1191–1216.

33a **Answer B.** Chondrosarcoma is a malignant tumor of the bone that produces chondroid matrix, characterized by mineralized rings and arcs as seen on the radiograph. These tumors exhibit a lobulated growth pattern with the lobules classically appearing hyperintense on fluid-sensitive sequences owing to the high water content in the hyaline cartilage.

Reference: Murphey MD, Walker EA, Wilson AJ, et al. From the archives of the AFIP: imaging of primary chondrosarcoma: radiologic-pathologic correlation. *Radiographics*. 2003;23(5):1245–1278.

33b **Answer C.** The lung is the most frequent site of metastatic disease. Other reported locations include the regional lymph nodes, liver, brain, and spine.

Reference: Murphey MD, Walker EA, Wilson AJ, et al. From the archives of the AFIP: imaging of primary chondrosarcoma: radiologic-pathologic correlation. *Radiographics*. 2003;23(5):1245–1278.

33c **Answer A.** Conventional chondrosarcomas occur most frequently in the femur and innominate bone. 10% to 20% of the cases occur in the upper extremity, primarily the proximal humerus. Other less common sites include tibia (5%), ribs (8%), spine (7%), scapula (5%), and sternum (2%).

References: Murphey MD, Walker EA, Wilson AJ, et al. From the archives of the AFIP: imaging of primary chondrosarcoma: radiologic-pathologic correlation. *Radiographics*. 2003;23(5):1245–1278.
Ozaki T, Hillmann A, Lindner N, Blasius S, et al. Metastasis of chondrosarcoma. *J Cancer Res Oncol*. 1996;122:625–628.

34 **Answer B.** Radiation induced osseous complications include chronic red marrow replacement, osteonecrosis, growth deformities, osteochondromas, and sarcomas. Radiation induced sarcomas are typically the complication of doses in the 5,000- to 6,000-cGy range, but have been reported as low as 2,000 to 3,000 cGy. The average latency period between therapy and sarcoma transformation is 11 years.

References: Lagrange J, Ramaioli A, Chateau M, et al. Sarcoma after radiation therapy: retrospective multi institutional study of 80 histologically confirmed cases. *Radiology.* 2000;216:197–205.

Manaster BJ, Roberts CC, Petersilge CA, et al. *Diagnostic Imaging: Musculoskeletal: Non-Traumatic Disease.* Manitoba, Canada: Amirsys; 2010;2:224–229.

35 **Answer B.** The imaging depicts Ewing sarcoma, a round cell sarcoma with a predilection for the diaphysis and metadiaphysis of long bones. A permeative, destructive osseous lesion with soft tissue mass is characteristic. The majority of cases occur in the pelvis, extremities, and ribs. Differential considerations include conventional osteosarcoma (high grade, intramedullary) and lymphoma, which has a permeative appearance and often a prominent soft tissue mass component. Following osteosarcoma, Ewing sarcoma is the most common primary, malignant bone tumor of childhood and adolescence.

Reference: Murphey MD, Senchak LT, Mambalam PK, et al. From the radiologic pathology archives: Ewing sarcoma family of tumors: radiologic-pathologic correlation. *Radiographics.* 2013;33:803–831.

36a **Answer B.** Langerhans cell histiocytosis is a neoplastic, clonal proliferation of histiocytes. Skin is the most common site of extraosseous disease involvement at 55%. In decreasing order of prevalence, additional extraosseous sites of disease manifestation include the central nervous system, hepatobiliary system and spleen, lungs, lymph nodes, soft tissues, bone marrow, salivary glands, and digestive tract.

References: Schmidt S, Eich G, Geoffray A, et al. Extraosseous Langerhans cell histiocytosis in children. *Radiographics.* 2008;28:707–726.

http://my.clevelandclinic.org/childrens-hospital/health-info/diseases-conditions/cancer/langerhans-cell-histiocytosis.aspx

36b **Answer A.** Although there is a wide reported mean age of diagnosis, the majority of Langerhans cell histiocytosis cases occur between 1 and 10 years of age.

References: Schmidt S, Eich G, Geoffray A, et al. Extraosseous Langerhans cell histiocytosis in children. *Radiographics.* 2008;28:707–726.

http://my.clevelandclinic.org/childrens-hospital/health-info/diseases-conditions/cancer/langerhans-cell-histiocytosis.aspx

37a **Answer B.** The lesion in the proximal radius is fibrous dysplasia. Tumor matrix is classified as chondroid, fibrous, or osseous. Fibrous dysplasia may be monostotic or polyostotic (15% to 20%). Typically lesions are located in the diaphysis but may extend into the metaphysis and epiphysis. Radiographic density may span the spectrum from lytic to sclerotic, but most have a ground-glass appearance. Lesions may cause varying degrees of bone expansion and bowing deformities.

Reference: Manaster BJ, May DA, Disler DG. *Musculoskeletal Imaging. The Requisites in Radiology.* 3rd ed. Philadelphia, PA: Elsevier; 2007:463.

37b **Answer C.** McCune-Albright syndrome is characterized by polyostotic fibrous dysplasia, endocrine abnormalities such as precocious puberty and hyperthyroidism, and café au lait skin lesions.

Reference: Manaster BJ, May DA, Disler DG. *Musculoskeletal Imaging. The Requisites in Radiology.* 3rd ed. Philadelphia, PA: Elsevier; 2007:463.

38 **Answer B.**   Radiographic and CT features of Paget disease in the pelvis and long bones include cortical and trabecular thickening, osseous enlargement, and osseous deformity.

Reference: Manaster BJ, Roberts CC, Petersilge CA, et al. *Diagnostic Imaging: Musculoskeletal: Non-Traumatic Disease*. Manitoba, Canada: Amirsys; 2010;2:184–186.

39a **Answer B.**   Myxomas are characteristically low to intermediate in signal intensity on T1-weighted and hyperintense on T2-weighted MR images. Intermediate to hypointense septations and nodularity are often present. Lesion enhancement is heterogeneous. The lesions are not associated with hemorrhage or hemosiderin deposition; thus, there is no blooming on T2* gradient-echo images.

References: Bancroft LW, Kransdorf MJ, Menke DM, et al. Intramuscular myxoma: characteristic MR imaging features. *AJR Am J Roentgenol*. 2002;178(5):1255–1259.
Manaster BJ, Roberts CC, Petersilge CA, et al. *Diagnostic Imaging: Musculoskeletal: Non-Traumatic Disease*. Manitoba, Canada: Amirsys; 2010;2:184–187.

39b **Answer C.**   Myxomas are intramuscular lesions most commonly located in the thigh, buttocks, and shoulder girdle.

References: Bancroft LW, Kransdorf MJ, Menke DM, et al. Intramuscular myxoma: characteristic MR imaging features. *AJR Am J Roentgenol*. 2002;178(5):1255–1259.
Manaster BJ, Roberts CC, Petersilge CA, et al. *Diagnostic Imaging: Musculoskeletal: Non-Traumatic Disease*. Manitoba, Canada: Amirsys; 2010;2:184–187.

39c **Answer A.**   Mazabraud syndrome is a combination of intramuscular myxomas and fibrous dysplasia.

References: Bancroft LW, Kransdorf MJ, Menke DM, et al. Intramuscular myxoma: characteristic MR imaging features. *AJR Am J Roentgenol*. 2002;178(5):1255–1259.
Manaster BJ, Roberts CC, Petersilge CA, et al. *Diagnostic Imaging: Musculoskeletal: Non-Traumatic Disease*. Manitoba, Canada: Amirsys; 2010;2:184–187.

40 **Answer D.**   Gorham disease (Gorham massive osteolysis, Gorham-Stout syndrome, disappearing bone disease) is a rare vascular disorder of lymphatic etiology characterized by spontaneous, progressive resorption of the bone. Gorham disease may affect any bone, although the skull, shoulder, and pelvis are most commonly involved. Osteolysis usually involves a single bone, but may extend to regional bones from a single focus, without regard for joint boundaries. Although a history of prior trauma is often elicited and pathologic fractures are not uncommon, these features are not specific for Gorham disease. Conversely, splenic lesions (cysts) and soft tissue changes adjacent to the site of skeletal involvement are commonly seen in patients with Gorham disease.

References: Kotecha R, Mascarenhas L, Jackson HA, et al. Radiological features of Gorham's disease. *Clin Radiol*. 2012;67(8):782–788.
Lala S, Mulliken JB, Alomari AI, et al. Gorham-Stout disease and generalized lymphatic anomaly – clinical, radiologic, and histologic differentiation. *Skeletal Radiol*. 2013;42:917–924.
Möller G, Priemel M, Amling M, et al. The Gorham-Stout syndrome (Gorham's massive osteolysis). A report of six cases with histopathological findings. *J Bone Joint Surg Br*. 2000;81(3):501–506.
Patel DV. Gorham's disease or massive osteolysis. *Clin Med Res*. 2005;3:65–74.

41a **Answer A.**   Radiographically, bone lesions should be described in detail to include their location, margin, zone of transition, periosteal reaction, mineralization/matrix, size, number of lesions, and presence/absence of a soft tissue component. Radiographically, this lesion in the proximal tibial metadiaphysis is best described as an eccentrically located lucent lesion with a distinct or geographic margin, thin peripheral sclerotic rim, and internal septations, descriptors all suggesting benignity. "Lucent" has a more benign connotation, whereas "lytic" suggests a more aggressive lesion. This lesion is not expansile and is not elongated and there are no aggressive features such as periosteal reaction, cortical breakthrough, soft tissue component, or pathologic fracture.

References: Levine SM, Lambiase RE, Petchprapa CN. Cortical lesions of the tibia: characteristic appearances at conventional radiography. *Radiographics.* 2003;23:157–177.
Miller TT. Bone tumors and tumorlike conditions: analysis with conventional radiography. *Radiology.* 2008;246;662–674.
Wilson AJ, Kyriakos M, Ackerman LV. Chondromyxoid fibroma: radiographic appearance in 38 cases and in a review of the literature. *Radiology.* 1991;179:513–518.

41b **Answer C.**   Chondromyxoid fibroma is a rare benign cartilaginous tumor of the bone, with approximately 50% of lesions developing in the tibia or femur. They are typically eccentrically located within the metaphysis with a geographic lobulated margin, septations, and a thin sclerotic rim, as seen in this case. They can also be elongated and expansile, and can erode through the cortex, but these features were not present in this case. Although chondromyxoid fibromas and aneurysmal bone cysts can have overlapping features, aneurysmal bone cysts are usually expansile with prominent cortical thinning, features that are not present in this case. Chondroblastoma is almost always an epiphyseal or apophyseal lesion. Eccentricity, internal septations, and thin sclerotic margin would be highly unusual features of osseous metastasis. Osteoblastomas are bone-producing tumors that most commonly occur in the axial skeleton. They are radiographically highly variable and may be blastic, lytic, or mixed lytic–blastic but often have a thick peripheral sclerosis similar to osteoid osteoma. The lesions may be well defined, exophytic, or very aggressive in radiographic appearance. Although a differential possibility in this location, choice E is not the most compatible choice for the radiographic and CT appearance of this lesion.

References: Levine SM, Lambiase RE, Petchprapa CN. Cortical lesions of the tibia: characteristic appearances at conventional radiography. *Radiographics.* 2003;23:157–177.
Miller TT. Bone tumors and tumorlike conditions: analysis with conventional radiography. *Radiology.* 2008;246;662–674.
Wilson AJ, Kyriakos M, Ackerman LV. Chondromyxoid fibroma: radiographic appearance in 38 cases and in a review of the literature. *Radiology.* 1991;179:513–518.

42 **Answer B.**   Bone island or enostosis is a focus of compact bone within the cancellous bone. They are homogeneously dense on radiographs and have a spiculated margin that blends with the adjacent bone. While bone islands are often cold or negative on bone scan, positive findings have been correlated histologically with bone islands. Sclerotic bone metastases are positive or hot on bone scan. Osteoblastomas are rare, benign bone tumors which may be lytic or contain variable amounts of mineralized matrix. They show intense uptake on bone scan. Multiple myeloma is characterized by lytic osseous lesions.

References: Greenspan A. Bone island (enostosis): current concept-a review. *Skeletal Radiol.* 1995;24(2):111–115.
Peh WCG, Muttarak M. Imaging in bone metastases. *Medscape (online reference).* March 8, 2013.

43 **Answer D.**   Osteoblastomas are bone-producing tumors that most commonly occur in the axial skeleton, but can occur in any bone in the body. They are radiographically highly variable and may be blastic, lytic, or mixed lytic–blastic, but often have a thick peripheral sclerosis similar to osteoid osteoma. The lesions may be well defined, exophytic, or very aggressive in radiographic appearance. Radiographically, the lesion in this case is best described as a metadiaphyseal, eccentric, geographic mixed lytic–blastic lesion with associated periosteal reaction in both the radius and ulna. Coronal CT shows an internal osteoid matrix and the periosteal reaction seen radiographically. Coronal proton density fat-saturated MR image shows prominent surrounding reactive marrow edema-like signal and adjacent soft tissue edema, typical of osteoblastoma. Although the radiographic appearance of osteoid osteoma and osteoblastoma can overlap, the size of this lesion favors osteoblastoma over osteoid osteoma. Chondroblastoma is an epiphyseal lesion that can have chondroid matrix, not osteoid matrix. Similarly, chondrosarcoma has chondroid matrix, not osteoid matrix. Also, the lack of a soft tissue mass component in the presence of prominent surrounding reactive inflammatory change makes chondrosarcoma unlikely. Osseous metastatic disease is overall unusual in children, and the surrounding sclerosis and osteoid matrix would be atypical findings; therefore, E is not the best choice.

Reference: Levine SM, Lambiase RE, Petchprapa CN. Cortical lesions of the tibia: characteristic appearances at conventional radiography. *Radiographics.* 2003;23:157–177.

44a **Answer B.**   Glomus tumor is a benign subungual tumor (hamartoma) developing from the neuromyoarterial glomus bodies. Thinning or erosion of the dorsal cortical bone of the distal phalanx may be seen radiographically. Glomus tumors typically demonstrate intermediate to low T1-weighted and high T2-weighted signal intensity relative to muscle. Because the glomus is richly vascularized, it shows marked contrast enhancement on MRI and MR angiography. Other possible diagnoses of a hypervascular subungual or periungual tumor are lobular capillary hemangioma (previously known as pyogenic granuloma) and true hemangioma. Melanomas are typically T1 hyperintense due to the presence of either melanin or hemorrhage. Giant cell tumors of the tendon sheath have nonspecific and variable T1 and T2 signal characteristics, but are more often low to intermediate on T2-weighted images. Contact with a tendon is also usually seen. Mucoid and epithelial inclusion cysts typically demonstrate thin peripheral rim enhancement, not homogeneous enhancement.

References: Baek HJ, Lee SJ, Cho KH, et al. Subungual tumors: clinicopathologic correlation with US and MR Imaging findings. *Radiographics.* 2010;30:1621–1636.
Hazani R, Houle JM, Kasdan ML. Glomus tumors of the hand. *Eplasty.* 2008;8:457–460.

44b **Answer D.**   Surgical excision is the treatment for glomus tumors, with complete resolution of symptoms following excision in all reported cases. No medical therapy exists.

References: Baek HJ, Lee SJ, Cho KH, et al. Subungual tumors: clinicopathologic correlation with US and MR imaging findings. *Radiographics.* 2010;30:1621–1636.
Hazani R, Houle JM, Kasdan ML. Glomus tumors of the hand. *Eplasty.* 2008;8:457–460.

45 **Answer C.**   The imaging findings demonstrate innumerable enchondromas involving the axial and appendicular skeleton with associated foci of mineralization in the soft tissues about the left knee, compatible with hemangiomas. The combination of enchondromas and hemangiomas is seen with Maffucci syndrome. There is loss of cortical definition and relative paucity of the chondroid matrix at the inferior aspect of the large chondroid lesion in the distal left femur with surrounding soft tissue prominence suggestive of a soft tissue mass component and worrisome for malignant transformation of an enchondroma to a secondary chondrosarcoma. These lesions do not resemble osteochondromas or nonossifying fibromas.

References: Bernard SA, Murphey MD, Flemming DJ, et al. Improved differentiation of benign osteochondromas from secondary chondrosarcomas with standardized measurement of cartilage cap on CT and MR imaging. *Radiology.* 2010;255:857–865.

Flach HZ, Ginai AZ, Oosterhuis JW. Best cases of the AFIP Maffucci syndrome: radiologic and pathologic findings. *Radiographics*. 2001;21:1311–1316.

Verdegaal SH, Bovee JV, Pansuriya TC, et al. Incidence, predictive factors, and prognosis of chondrosarcoma in patients with Ollier disease and Maffucci syndrome: an international multicenter study of 161 patients. *Oncologist*. 2011;16(12):1771–1779.

46 **Answer B.**   The mass is diffusely and avidly enhancing, has intimate association with the tendons of the thumb, and has associated underlying bony erosion, all of which support the diagnosis of giant cell tumor of the tendon sheath, which is the second most common soft tissue mass in the hand and wrist. Although a ganglion is the most common soft tissue mass in the hand and wrist, it typically demonstrates thin peripheral enhancement on postcontrast imaging. Hemangioma can demonstrate diffuse avid enhancement as seen in this case, but the lack of associated internal fat and phleboliths make this diagnosis less likely. These MRI findings are not typical of infection given the lack of surrounding soft tissue inflammatory change and the lack of underlying marrow signal change in the presence of bone erosion.

Reference: Teh J, Whiteley G. MRI of soft tissue masses of the hand and wrist. *Br J Radiol*. 2007;80:47–63.

47 **Answer C.**   Parosteal osteosarcoma is a densely ossified juxtacortical mass that lies outside the cortex and occurs in the metaphyses. In contrast to osteochondroma, parosteal osteosarcoma lacks corticomedullary continuity between the tumor and the underlying medullary canal. There is no corticomedullary continuity associated with the mass in this case. The ossification pattern of parosteal osteosarcoma is the radiographic inverse of that seen in myositis ossificans. In myositis ossificans, the most dense bone is typically seen in the periphery, whereas in parosteal osteosarcoma, the most dense bone is seen centrally, with the least radiopaque bone at the periphery. On MRI, there is usually prominent soft tissue edema surrounding myositis ossificans, which would be unusual in parosteal osteosarcoma. Periosteal chondromas are typically metaphyseal in location and commonly present on radiographs as lucent juxtacortical lesions with variable degrees of chondroid matrix calcifications. They can cause cortical saucerization with a well-formed periosteal reaction, features not associated with parosteal osteosarcoma. At MR imaging, periosteal chondromas are T2 hyperintense, whereas parosteal osteosarcoma is typically hypointense on T1- and T2-weighted images due to dense ossification. Unlike parosteal osteosarcoma, periosteal osteosarcoma is usually more lytic in appearance, causes cortical erosion and periosteal reaction, and occurs in diaphyses.

Reference: Yarmish G, Klein MJ, Landa J, et al. Imaging characteristics of primary osteosarcoma: nonconventional subtypes. *Radiographics*. 2010;30:1653–1672.

48 **Answer B.**   Telangiectatic osteosarcoma is a rare variant of osteogenic sarcoma consisting of large hemorrhagic or necrotic spaces surrounded by viable sarcomatous tissue. Fluid-filled cavities make up the majority of such tumors (>90%). Internal fluid–fluid levels are commonly seen on CT and MRI, although such findings are not specific to telangiectatic osteosarcoma. Fluid–fluid levels are also characteristically seen with aneurysmal bone cysts (ABC), which are benign tumor-like lesions of the bone. Because prognosis and treatment of these two entities differ substantially, accurate diagnosis is imperative. Imaging features that favor telangiectatic osteosarcoma over ABC include

1. Thick nodular septations and a surrounding soft tissue component (best demonstrated on CT or MRI following contrast administration)
2. Matrix mineralization in the lesion
3. Cortical destruction or other aggressive features

In the case presented, there is clear evidence of cortical destruction along the lateral margin of the lesion indicating an aggressive behavior. On the provided T2-weighted fat-saturated MR image, only thin septations are evident. Expansile remodeling is more typical of a slow-growing nonaggressive lesion such as ABC. Both telangiectatic osteosarcoma and ABC may be eccentrically located.

References: Discepola F, Powell TI, Nahal A. Telangiectatic osteosarcoma: radiologic and pathologic findings. *Radiographics* 2009;29:380–383.

Murphey MD, wan Jaovishidha S, Temple HT, et al. Telangiectatic osteosarcoma: radiologic-pathologic correlation. *Radiology.* 2003;229:549–553.

49   **Answer C.**   Pigmented villonodular synovitis (PVNS) is a rare benign neoplasm arising from synovial tissue. Hemosiderin deposition within hypertrophied synovial tissue is seen in the majority of cases. On MRI, hemosiderin shortens the T2 relaxation time accounting for the pathognomonic low signal intensity of PVNS on T2-weighted sequences. Magnetic field inhomogeneities associated with hemosiderin are accentuated on gradient-echo sequences, with faster T2* relaxation leading to further loss of signal intensity. This phenomenon is typically referred to as blooming.

References: Chavhan GB, Babyn PS, Thomas B, et al. Principles, techniques, and applications of T2*-based MR imaging and its special applications. *Radiographics.* 2009;29(5):1433–1449.

Murphey MD, Rhee JH, Lewis RB, et al. Pigmented villonodular synovitis: radiologic-pathologic correlation. *Radiographics.* 2008;28:1493–1518.

50   **Answer A.**   Chondroblastoma is an uncommon neoplasm of chondroid origin that typically arises in the epiphysis or apophysis of long bones in skeletally immature patients. Although the location and radiographic appearance of chondroblastoma are often diagnostic, MRI may allow for a more confident diagnosis in cases where atypical features are encountered. Extensive bone marrow edema surrounding an otherwise well-circumscribed epiphyseal lesion in a skeletally immature patient is highly characteristic of chondroblastoma. Such edema should not be misinterpreted as indicating a more aggressive process such as infection or malignant neoplasm.

References: Kaim AH, Hugli R, Bonel HM, et al. Chondroblastoma and clear cell chondrosarcoma: radiological and MRI characteristics with histopathological correlation. *Skeletal Radiol.* 2002;31:88–95.

Weatherall PT, Maale GE, Mendelsohn DB, et al. Chondroblastoma: classic and confusing appearance at MR imaging. *Radiology.* 1994;190:467–474.

51   **Answer A.**   Angiosarcoma of the bone is a rare high-grade malignant tumor of vascular origin. Local recurrence and distant metastases are common with overall poor survival. Identification of serpentine vascular channels within an aggressive appearing tumor should suggest the diagnosis. Prominent vascular channels would be rare in other tumors including lymphoma, plasmacytoma, and sarcomas of nonvascular origin. In contrast to hemangiomas, these tumors are not associated with fatty overgrowth and demonstrate aggressive features including infiltration of the surrounding tissues. In the case presented, multifocal areas of tangled vascular channels are evident within an aggressive appearing lesion making answer A (angiosarcoma) the most likely diagnosis.

References: Murphey MD, Fairbairn KJ, Parman LM, et al. Musculoskeletal angiomatous lesions: radiologic-pathologic correlation. *Radiographics.* 1995;15(4):893–917.

Palmerini E, Maki RG, Staals EL, et al. Primary angiosarcoma of bone. A retrospective analysis of 60 patients from 2 institutions. *Am J Clin Oncol.* [Epub ahead of print], 2013.

52   **Answer C.**   Lipoma arborescens is a rare, benign intra-articular process characterized by lipomatous proliferation of the synovial capsule. The suprapatellar pouch of the knee is the most common site of involvement. The etiology of lipoma arborescens is unclear, although this entity is often seen in association with underlying chronic joint pathology. MR allows for an accurate diagnosis by demonstrating a frond-like synovial mass keeping with fat signal intensity on all imaging sequences. In the images provided, there is synovial proliferation with conspicuous fat signal intensity on both T1-weighted and T2-weighted fat-saturated images.

References: Bancroft LW, Kransdorf MJ, Peterson JJ, et al. Benign fatty tumors: classification, clinical course, imaging appearance, and treatment. *Skeletal Radiol.* 2006;35:719–733.
Ryu KN, Jaovisidha S, Schweitzer M, et al. MR imaging of lipoma arborescens of the knee joint. *AJR Am J Roentgenol.* 1996;167:1229–1232.
Vilanova JC, Barcelo J, Villalon M, et al. MR imaging of lipoma arborescens and associated lesions. *Skeletal Radiol.* 2003;32:504–509.

53a Answer D.   Periosteal reaction occurs in response to a wide variety of osseous insults. Multiple patterns of periosteal new bone formation may occur, often with considerable overlap of appearance in benign and malignant lesions. In general, periosteal reaction may be classified as nonaggressive or aggressive in appearance. Nonaggressive patterns of periosteal reaction include thin, thick, solid, thick irregular, and septated varieties. These types of periosteal reaction are typically seen with benign, slow processes such as healing fractures or osteoid osteoma. Aggressive forms of periosteal reaction include laminated or lamellated (onion skin), spiculated (perpendicular or sunburst), disorganized, and marginal periosteal elevation (Codman triangle). Such patterns of periosteal reaction suggest a more aggressive biologic behavior and can be seen in the setting of primary bone tumors, infection, and metastases. In the present case, spicules of periosteal new bone radiate from the femoral shaft in a divergent pattern typical of an aggressive spiculated (sunburst)-type pattern.

References: Miller TT. Bone tumors and tumorlike conditions: analysis with conventional radiography. *Radiology.* 2008;246(3):662–674.
Rana RS, Wu JS, Eisenberg RL. Periosteal reaction. *AJR Am J Roentgenol* 2009;193(4): W259–W272.

53b Answer C.   Of the entities presented, choice C (conventional osteosarcoma) is most likely to demonstrate a spiculated (sunburst) type of periosteal reaction. Osteomyelitis may also demonstrate a spiculated pattern of periosteal reaction, although more commonly is characterized as disorganized, thin, or lamellated. Eosinophilic granuloma lesions may be associated with a thick or laminated pattern of periosteal reaction, especially during the healing phase. Periosteal reaction associated with chondroblastoma most commonly occurs in large lesions and can be thick, solid, or laminated.

References: Miller TT. Bone tumors and tumorlike conditions: analysis with conventional radiography. *Radiology.* 2008;246(3):662–674.
Rana RS, Wu JS, Eisenberg RL. Periosteal reaction. *AJR Am J Roentgenol* 2009;193(4): W259–W272.

54 Answer C.   The prognosis for parosteal osteosarcoma is better than that for periosteal osteosarcoma, high grade surface osteosarcoma, conventional osteosarcoma, and telangiectatic osteosarcoma. The 5-year overall survival rate is 86% to 91% for parosteal osteosarcoma, 83% for periosteal osteosarcoma, 67% for telangiectatic osteosarcoma, and 53% to 61% for conventional osteosarcoma. The reported 5-year survival rate for high-grade surface osteosarcoma is 46.1%.

Reference: Yarmish G, Klein MJ, Landa J, et al. Imaging characteristics of primary osteosarcoma: nonconventional subtypes. *Radiographics.* 2010;30:1653–1672.

55 Answer A.   The rate of malignant transformation of enchondromas into chondrosarcoma or fibrosarcoma in Maffucci syndrome varies between 15% and 56%. In Ollier disease, the rate of malignant transformation of the skeletal lesions is 25% to 30%. A more recent study of 161 patients including those with Ollier disease (*n* = 144) and Maffucci syndrome (*n* = 17) found an overall incidence of malignant transformation to chondrosarcoma of 40%. The prevalence of malignant transformation of osteochondroma in the setting of multiple hereditary exostoses is 2% to 5%. Malignant transformation of nonossifying fibromas in Jaffe-Campanacci syndrome and of osteomas in Gardner syndrome has not been reported.

References: Bernard SA, Murphey MD, Flemming DJ, et al. Improved differentiation of benign osteochondromas from secondary chondrosarcomas with standardized measurement of cartilage cap on CT and MR imaging. *Radiology.* 2010;255:857–865.

Flach HZ, Ginai AZ, Oosterhuis JW. Best cases of the AFIP Maffucci syndrome: radiologic and pathologic findings. *Radiographics.* 2001;21:1311–1316.

Verdegaal SH, Bovee JV, Pansuriya TC, et al. Incidence, predictive factors, and prognosis of chondrosarcoma in patients with Ollier disease and Maffucci syndrome: an international multicenter study of 161 patients. *Oncologist.* 2011;16(12):1771–1779.

56 Answer C. Phleboliths are commonly seen on radiographs in association with hemangiomas. Phleboliths are not associated with giant cell tumor of the tendon sheath. Hemangiomas are soft tissues masses, but the identification of a soft tissue mass alone on a radiograph would not serve to narrow the differential diagnosis. Bony erosion and cortical thickening are not typically associated with soft tissue hemangiomas in the hand.

Reference: Teh J, Whiteley G. MRI of soft tissue masses of the hand and wrist. *Br J Radiol.* 2007;80:47–63.

57 Answer B. Osteosarcoma (osteogenic sarcoma) is the most common primary malignant bone tumor in children and adolescents. 5% to 10% of cases have pulmonary metastatic disease at the time of diagnosis. Most cases occur in patients in their second and third decades with a slight male predominance. The vast majority of osteosarcomas arise in the metaphysis of long bones. Of all of the variants of osteosarcoma, conventional osteosarcoma accounts for approximately 75% of cases.

Reference: Murphey MD, Robbin MR, McRae GA, et al. The many faces of osteosarcoma. *Radiographics.* 1997;17(5):1205–1231.

58 Answer A. Malignant fibrous histiocytoma (MFH) is a pleomorphic sarcoma that occurs most commonly in soft tissues, although it may also occur primarily in bone. MFH of the bone accounts for 5% of all primary malignant bone tumors with a peak prevalence in the fourth decade of life. Most tumors arise in the appendicular skeleton, predominantly centered in the metaphysis of long tubular bones. Although most cases of MFH arise spontaneously, tumors can also develop in the setting of prior radiation, surgery, trauma, or preexisting benign osseous lesions. In contrast to other primary tumors of the bone, MFH is not typically associated with periosteal reaction. It generally does not have a sclerotic margin and does have an associated soft tissue mass, findings consistent with malignancy. It typically does not have cortical expansion.

References: Murphey MD, Gross TM, Rosenthal HG. From the archives of the AFIP: musculoskeletal malignant fibrous histiocytoma: radiologic-pathologic correlation. *Radiographics.* 1994;14(4):807–826.

Ros PR, Viamonte M, Rywlin AM. Malignant fibrous histiocytoma: mesenchymal tumor of ubiquitous origin. *AJR Am J Roentgenol.* 1984;142:753–759.

59a Answer C. Nodular fasciitis is a benign fibrous proliferation, which may be mistaken for sarcoma given its rapid growth and high cellularity. The majority of lesions are located in the upper extremities with the trunk, head and neck, and lower extremities being less common. Most commonly, nodular fasciitis is subcutaneous, fascial based, and well circumscribed. Intramuscular and para-articular locations have been described, in addition to transcompartmental spread and osseous invasion.

References: Coyle J, White LM, Dickson B, et al. MRI characteristics of nodular fasciitis of the musculoskeletal system. *Skeletal Radiol.* 2013;42(7):975–982.

Dinauer PA, Brixey CJ, Moncur JT, et al. Pathologic and MR imaging features of benign fibrous soft-tissue tumors in adults. *Radiographics.* 2007;27:173–187.

59b Answer A.   Nodular fasciitis has a self-limited course, and both marginal surgical excision and observation only are acceptable treatment options.

References: Coyle J, White LM, Dickson B, et al. MRI characteristics of nodular fasciitis of the musculoskeletal system. *Skeletal Radiol.* 2013;42(7):975–982.

Dinauer PA, Brixey CJ, Moncur JT, et al. Pathologic and MR imaging features of benign fibrous soft-tissue tumors in adults. *Radiographics.* 2007;27:173–187.

60 Answer A.   Adamantinoma is a rare, low-grade osseous malignancy that has a predilection for the anterior cortex of the tibial diaphysis. Fibular cases have also been reported. It is expansile, multilocular with areas of sclerosis and lysis, and has a narrow zone of transition. Cortical breakthrough occurs in 15% to 50% of cases. Soft tissue mass and solid periosteal reaction are associated with cortical breakthrough.

References: Camp MD, Tompkins RK, Spanier SS, et al. Adamantinoma of the tibia and fibula with cytogenetic analysis. *Radiographics.* 2008;28:1215–1220.

Manaster BJ, Roberts CC, Petersilge CA, et al. *Diagnostic Imaging: Musculoskeletal: Non-Traumatic Disease.* Manitoba, Canada: Amirsys; 2010;2:164–167.

61a Answer A.   The MRI is an example of a well-differentiated liposarcoma (atypical lipomatous tumor). The World Health Organization Committee on Classification of Soft Tissue Tumors has designated these terms as being synonymous. The lesion is composed of fat, but has mildly thick septations, mild heterogeneity on T2 weighted images, and mild lesional enhancement. There were no myxoid or nonfatty, solid components.

References: Gaskin CM, Helms CA. Lipomas, lipoma variants, and well-differentiated liposarcomas (atypical lipomas): results of MRI evaluations of 126 consecutive fatty masses. *AJR Am J Roentgenol.* 2004;182:733–739.

Murphey MD, Arcara LK, Fanburg-Smith J. Imaging of musculoskeletal liposarcoma with radiologic-pathologic correlation. *Radiographics.* 2005;25:1371–1395.

61b Answer A.   Following surgical excision of an extremity lesion, local surveillance is recommended. Well-differentiated liposarcomas may recur locally but, in the absence of dedifferentiation, have no metastatic potential.

References: Gaskin CM, Helms CA. Lipomas, lipoma variants, and well-differentiated liposarcomas (atypical lipomas): results of MRI evaluations of 126 consecutive fatty masses. *AJR Am J Roentgenol.* 2004;182:733–739.

Murphey MD, Arcara LK, Fanburg-Smith J. Imaging of musculoskeletal liposarcoma with radiologic-pathologic correlation. *Radiographics.* 2005;25:1371–1395.

62 Answer C.   Imaging is not a reliable tool for the determination of lesion grade. If the lesion does not have a pathognomonic appearance of a specific, benign entity, for instance lipoma, hemangioma, or schwannoma, it should be considered malignant. Of the options, the appropriate next step in diagnosing a malignant soft tissue tumor is biopsy.

References: Manaster BJ, Roberts CC, Petersilge CA, et al. *Diagnostic Imaging: Musculoskeletal: Non-Traumatic Disease.* Manitoba, Canada: Amirsys; 2010;3:2.

Wu JS, Hochman MG. Soft-tissue tumors and tumorlike lesions: a systematic imaging approach. *Radiology.* 2009;253:297–316.

63 **Answer B.** The images depict an aneurysmal bone cyst in the patella. The lesion is hyperintense on T2-weighted images with septal enhancement following contrast administration. Fluid–fluid levels are evident. The majority of primary patellar tumors are benign with chondroblastoma and giant cell tumor being most common.

References: Kransdorf MJ, Moser RP, Vinh TN, et al. Primary tumors of the patella. A review of 42 cases. *Skeletal Radiol.* 1989;18(5):365–371.

Singh J, James SL, Kroon HM, et al. Tumour and tumour-like lesions of the patella – a multicentre experience. Eur Radiol. 2009;19:701–712.

64 **Answer C.** Hemangioendotheliomas, along with Kaposi sarcoma and angiosarcoma, are vascular sarcomas arising from endothelial cells or their precursors. Hemangioendotheliomas are generally less aggressive than angiosarcomas. Leiomyosarcoma is a tumor arising from smooth muscle cells of blood vessels. Polycythemia vera is a myeloproliferative disorder of uncontrolled red blood cell production.

Reference: Cioffi A, Reichert S, Antonescu CR, et al. Angiosarcomas and other sarcomas of endothelial origin. *Hematol Oncol Clin N Am.* 2013;27:975–988.

65 **Answer D.** The images are of multiple myeloma, a plasma cell disorder of the bone marrow. It is the most common primary bone malignancy characterized by lytic lesions. Epidural disease spread is common; extramedullary disease is uncommon. Sclerotic multiple myeloma is rare and associated with POEMS syndrome (polyneuropathy, organomegaly, endocrinopathy, M-protein, skin lesions). Differential considerations for lytic bone lesions include metastases, lymphoma, and leukemia. Osteoporosis is a reduction in the histologically normal bone. Lymphangioma is a soft tissue lesion composed of dilated lymphatic channels. Prostate metastases are characteristically blastic.

References: Manaster BJ, Roberts CC, Petersilge CA, et al. *Diagnostic Imaging: Musculoskeletal: Non-Traumatic Disease.* Manitoba, Canada: Amirsys; 2010;2:114–119.

Walker RC, Brown TL, Jones-Jackson LB, et al. Imaging of multiple myeloma and related plasma cell dyscrasias. *J Nucl Med.* 2012;53(7):1091–1101.

66 **Answer D.** The radiograph and MR images depict a periosteal chondroma (synonym: juxtacortical chondroma), which is a benign, cartilage tumor arising on the surface of the bone deep to the periosteum. They have a predilection for the metaphysis of long bones. Radiographically, the lesion causes saucerization of the cortex with sclerotic margination and dense periosteal reaction along the proximal and distal ends of the lesion. Lesion matrix mineralization is present in approximately 75% of cases. The lesions are hypointense on T1-weighted and hyperintense on T2-weighted MR images, owing to the chondroid composition. The lesions are rare, accounting for <2% of all chondromas.

References: Manaster BJ, Roberts CC, Petersilge CA, et al. *Diagnostic Imaging: Musculoskeletal: Non-Traumatic Disease.* Manitoba, Canada: Amirsys; 2010;3:94–99.

Woertler K, Blasius S, Brinkschmidt C, et al. Periosteal chondroma: MR characteristics. *J Comput Assist Tomogr.* 2001;25(3):425–430.

67 **Answer A.** The term hemangiopericytoma was originally described as a distinct vascular tumor with a staghorn-branching vascular pattern. This pattern is now characterized as a histopathologic pattern rather than a distinct clinicopathologic entity, and the term solitary fibrous tumor is favored by soft tissue pathologists. However, the terms hemangiopericytoma and solitary fibrous tumor are used interchangeably by some authors. Solitary fibrous tumor is a heterogeneous group of benign and malignant neoplasms composed of spindle cells. Oncogenic hypoglycemia and osteomalacia have been associated with these lesions.

References: Cho S, Do N, Yu S, et al. Nasal hemangiopericytoma causing oncogenic osteomalacia. *Clin Exp Otorhinolaryngol.* 2012;5(3):173–176.
Murphey MD, Fairbairn KJ, Parman LM, et al. From the archives of the AFIP: musculoskeletal angiomatous lesions: radiologic-pathologic correlation. *Radiographics.* 1995;15:893–917.
Penel N, Amela EY, Decanter G, et al. Solitary fibrous tumors and so-called hemangiopericytoma. *Sarcoma.* 2012;2012:690251.

68 Answer A.   The correct approach to a lesion in the proximal tibial metaphysis is anteromedial. This pathway avoids traversing musculature and contaminating the popliteal vasculature or tibial nerve. Tumor seeding of the biopsy tract has been shown to cause local recurrence of bone sarcomas; thus, the biopsy tract is resected by the surgeon. An incorrect tract may necessitate a more complex surgery or enlarge the radiation field. Teaching point: Always biopsy in the plane of surgical resection.

Reference: Liu PT, Valadez SD, Chivers FS, et al. Anatomically based guidelines for core needle biopsy of bone tumors: implications for limb-sparing surgery. *Radiographics.* 2007;27:189–205.

69 Answer C.   Periosteal osteosarcoma is an intermediate-grade surface neoplasm. In 68% of cases, calcified spicules of the bone extending perpendicular to the cortical margin will be visible radiographically. Characteristically, bone formation is denser near the cortical margin with a soft tissue mass extending from the tumor osteoid. Marrow involvement is rare. Conversely, imaging of parosteal osteosarcomas classically shows a surface soft tissue mass with mature bone extending from the center of the lesion to the periphery with the marrow nearly always involved.

References: Manaster BJ, Roberts CC, Petersilge CA, et al. *Diagnostic Imaging: Musculoskeletal: Non-Traumatic Disease.* Manitoba, Canada: Amirsys; 2010;2:44–53.
Murphey MD, Jelinek JS, Temple HT, et al. Imaging of periosteal osteosarcoma: radiologic-pathologic comparison. *Radiology.* 2004;233:129–138.

70 Answer B.   The condition described is cystic angiomatosis. Radiographically, the lesions are characteristically round or ovoid, well defined, and lytic with sclerotic margins with no matrix formation or periosteal reaction. Visceral organ involvement is present in 60% to 70% of cases.

References: Boyse TD, Jacobson JA. Case 45: cystic angiomatosis. *Radiology.* 2002;223:164–167.
Levey DS, MacCormack LM, Sartoris DJ, et al. Cystic angiomatosis: case report and review of the literature. *Skeletal Radiol.* 1996;25(3):287–293.

71 Answer D.   The lesion in the humerus is best described as an ill-defined, lytic lesion with a permeative pattern of osseous destruction (type 3 margin). This margin is characteristic of an aggressive bone lesion/process such as lymphoma, osteosarcoma, Ewing sarcoma, and osteomyelitis. This case is an example of osseous lymphoma. Answer A describes a type 1b margin, and answer C describes a type 1c margin. Answer B is not a correct margin description.

Reference: Miller TT. Bone tumors and tumorlike conditions: analysis with conventional radiography. *Radiology.* 2008;246:662–674.

72 Answer A.   The radiograph shows a lytic lesion in the distal radius with associated pathologic fracturing. The best primary tumor is renal cell carcinoma (RCC). Bone metastases have been reported to occur in approximately 30% of patients with RCC. Metastatic lesions in RCC are typically expansile, lytic, and hypervascular. Neuroblastoma is a tumor of childhood, most commonly affecting those 5 years and younger. Blastic, not lytic, metastases are typical for prostate carcinoma. Lytic metastasis may be seen in papillary thyroid carcinoma, although uncommon (1% to 7%).

References: Durante C, Haddy N, Baudin E, et al. Long-term outcome of 444 patients with distant metastases from papillary and follicular thyroid carcinoma: benefits and limits of radioiodine therapy. *J Clin Endocrinol Metab.* 2006;91:2892–2899.

Lipton A, Colombo-Berra A, Bukowski RM, et al. Skeletal complications in patients with bone metastases from renal cell carcinoma and therapeutic benefits of zoledronic acid. *Clin Cancer Res.* 2004;10:6397S.

Setlik DE, McCluskey KM, McDavit JA. Renal cell carcinoma manifesting as a solitary bone metastasis. *Radiographics.* 2009;29:2184–2189.

73 **Answer D.** Osseous lymphoma arises in the location of persistent red marrow with a peak incidence in the sixth and seventh decades of life. The lesion is lytic with permeative bone destruction and no true matrix. Periosteal reaction is present in approximately 60% of cases. Cortical destruction is often subtle, if at all visible, radiographically. A soft tissue mass is characteristic, and it may be small or disproportionately large.

Reference: Manaster BJ, Roberts CC, Petersilge CA, et al. *Diagnostic Imaging: Musculoskeletal: Non-Traumatic Disease.* Manitoba, Canada: Amirsys; 2010;2I:132–137.

74 **Answer C.** The imaged lesion is a desmoid tumor (desmoid-type fibromatosis, extra-abdominal desmoid, aggressive fibromatosis). Desmoid tumors are nonmetastasizing, ill-defined, infiltrative masses, which are locally aggressive. Skeletal maturation has no bearing on their growth potential, and calcification or ossification is rare. Local recurrence ranges from approximately 19% to 77%. Lesions are often debilitating and may be fatal due to invasion of local structures. Wide, local surgical excision, radiotherapy, and chemotherapy have been used as treatments.

References: Lee JC, Thomas M, Phillips S, et al. Aggressive fibromatosis: MRI features with pathologic correlation. *AJR Am J Roentgenol.* 2006;186:247–254.

Shinagare AB, Ramaiya NH, Jagannathan JP, et al. A to Z of desmoid tumors. *AJR Am J Roentgenol.* 2011;197:W1008–W1014.

75 **Answer D.** There is considerable imaging overlap between the types of soft tissue sarcomas, and thus tissue diagnosis is essential. Malignant fibrous histiocytoma (undifferentiated pleomorphic sarcoma) is the most common accounting for approximately 24% of soft tissue sarcomas.

Reference: Kransdorf MJ, Murphey MD. *Imaging of Soft Tissue Tumors.* 2nd ed. Philadelphia, PA: Lippincott Williams & Wilkins; 2006:6–37, 80–149.

1 What injury mechanism produces the soft tissue and osseous findings depicted below?

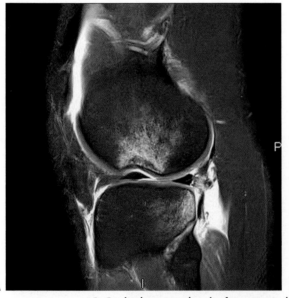 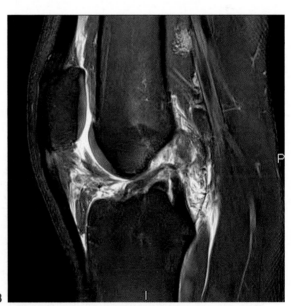

A **A.** Sagittal proton density fat saturated **B.** Sagittal proton density fat saturated B

A. Pivot shift
B. Hyperextension
C. Clipping
D. Dashboard

2 Which of the following correctly matches the extensor tendon with its appropriate dorsal wrist compartment?

A. Extensor pollicis longus—compartment I
B. Abductor pollicis longus—compartment II
C. Extensor indicis—compartment III
D. Extensor carpi ulnaris—compartment IV
E. Extensor digiti minimi—compartment V

3   In the setting of the following injury, what is the next most appropriate imaging study?

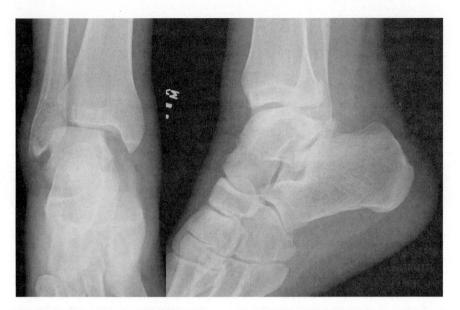

A. Stress radiographs of the ankle
B. Tibia/fibula radiographs
C. Ankle MRI
D. Ankle CT

4a   Axial and oblique sagittal MR images of the shoulder are provided. The imaged paralabral cyst is located within what anatomic space?

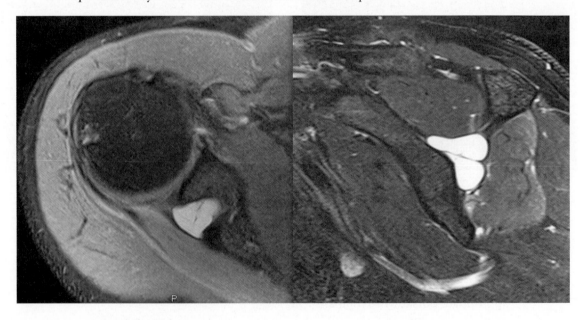

A. Quadrilateral space
B. Suprascapular notch
C. Rotator interval
D. Spinoglenoid notch

4b Compression of the suprascapular nerve in the spinoglenoid notch classically results in denervation of what muscle or muscles?

A. Supraspinatus
B. Supraspinatus and infraspinatus
C. Infraspinatus
D. Teres minor
E. Teres minor and deltoid

5 Coronal and sagittal T1-weighted images of the wrist are provided. What wrist abnormality is frequented associated with the imaged pathology?

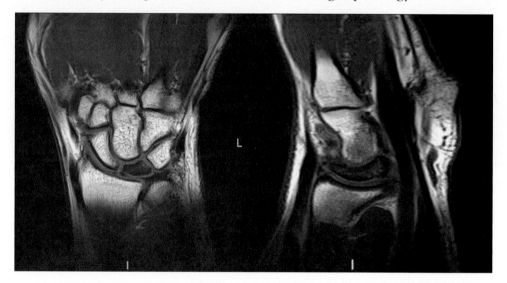

A. Ulnar positive variance
B. Lunotriquetral coalition
C. Ulnar negative variance
D. Distal radioulnar impingement

6 A 32-year-old male presented 18 months after surgery with the following CT scan. What is the most likely diagnosis?

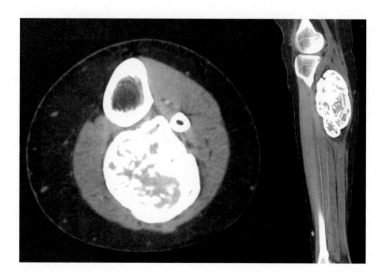

A. Heterotopic ossification
B. Parosteal osteosarcoma
C. Tumoral calcinosis
D. Osteochondroma

7a Axial and sagittal T2-weighted fat-suppressed images of the elbow are provided. The images depict what abnormality?

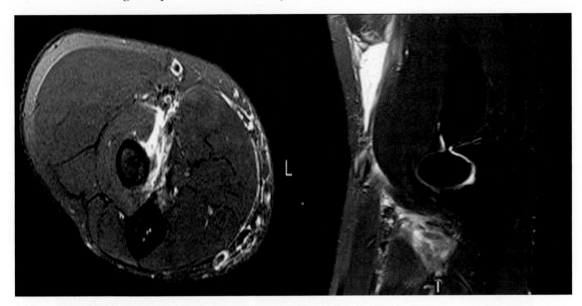

    A. Bicipitoradial bursitis
    B. Brachialis tendon tear
    C. Biceps tendon tear
    D. Cephalic vein thrombus

7b What structure can prevent proximal retraction of the biceps tendon, even if complete disruption of the tendon has occurred?

    A. Biceps tendon sheath
    B. Brachialis tendon
    C. Lacertus fibrosis
    D. Bicipitoradial bursa

8 The provided image demonstrates avulsion of what tendinous insertion?

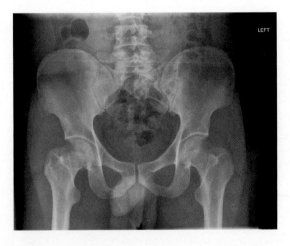

    A. Rectus femoris
    B. Gluteus medius
    C. Iliopsoas
    D. Rectus abdominis
    E. Sartorius

9   Radiographs of the right forearm demonstrate a combination of injuries that are commonly referred to as

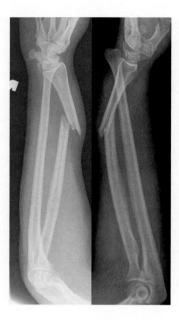

A. Monteggia fracture.
B. Galeazzi fracture.
C. Essex-Lopresti fracture.
D. Barton fracture.
E. Smith fracture.

10   What is the most common cause of posterior shoulder dislocation in adult patients?

A. Fall on outstretched hand
B. Direct posterior blow
C. Iatrogenic
D. Seizure

11   A lateral radiograph of the right foot is provided. These findings are concerning for injury to the ligament that spans what space?

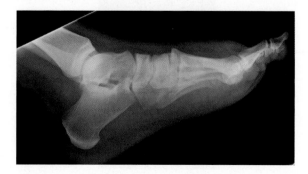

A. Lateral cuneiform and fifth metatarsal base
B. Intermediate cuneiform and first metatarsal base
C. Medial cuneiform and second metatarsal base
D. Medial and intermediate cuneiforms

12   A cross-table lateral view of the left knee is provided. Further imaging should be performed primarily to exclude which of the following abnormalities?

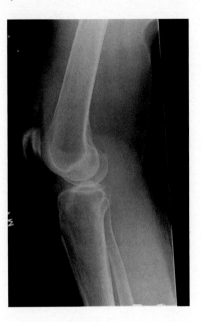

    A. Anterior cruciate ligament injury
    B. Occult fracture
    C. Lateral patellar dislocation
    D. Medial meniscus tear

13   A patient presents to the emergency department with acute foot pain following a sports injury. Based on the radiograph below, what is the best diagnosis?

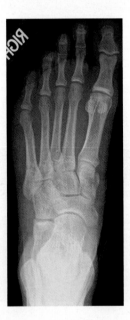

    A. Jones fracture
    B. Fifth metatarsal base avulsion fracture
    C. Proximal diaphyseal stress fracture
    D. Salter-Harris type 1 fracture
    E. Salter-Harris type 2 fracture

◦ . **14** The imaged pathology affects which of the following extensor tendons?

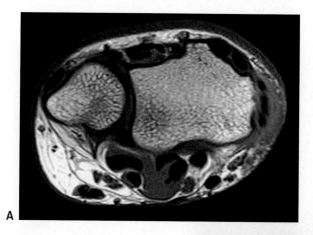

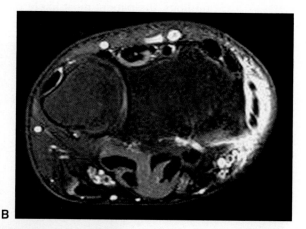

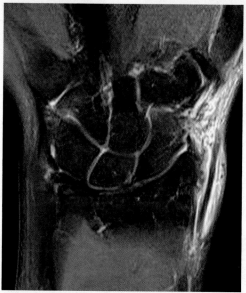

A. Axial T1 weighted **B.** Axial T2 weighted fat saturated **C.** Coronal T2 weighted fat saturated

    A. Extensor carpi radialis brevis
    B. Extensor pollicis longus
    C. Extensor carpi ulnaris
    D. Extensor digitorum
    E. Extensor pollicis brevis

15 Anterior "kissing contusions" in the knee are seen with which of the following injury mechanisms?

    A. Pivot shift
    B. Dashboard
    C. Hyperextension
    D. Clipping
    E. Lateral patellar dislocation

16 The following patient presented with shoulder pain. Based on the imaging findings, the patient most likely participates in which of the following activities?

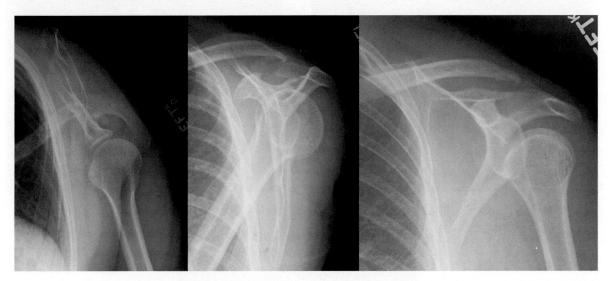

    A. Baseball pitching
    B. Weight lifting
    C. American football
    D. Gymnastics

17 A 20-year-old male presents to the emergency department complaining of hand pain and swelling after a fall. Which of the following statements is true regarding his condition?

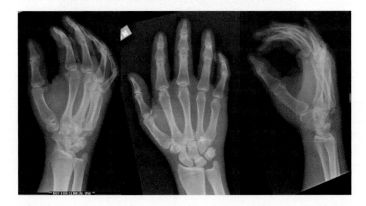

    A. There is a high association with metacarpophalangeal dislocation.
    B. Carpometacarpal dislocation without fracture is rare.
    C. Carpometacarpal dislocation most commonly occurs volarly.
    D. One view is usually sufficient to make the diagnosis.

18 Which pattern of dislocation most commonly occurs at the glenohumeral joint?
    A. Anterior infracoracoid
    B. Anterior subglenoid
    C. Intrathoracic
    D. Posterior

19 An 18-year-old male has an MRI performed after an acute kicking injury and right hip pain. What is the diagnosis?

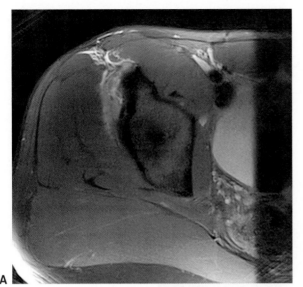 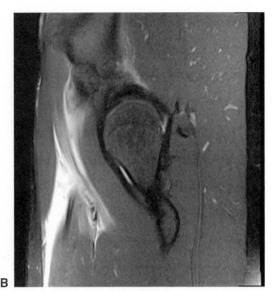

A   B

A. Axial T2 weighted fat saturated **B.** Sagittal T2 weighted fat saturated

    A. Stress fracture
    B. Acetabular labral tear
    C. Sartorius tendon tear
    D. Rectus femoris tendon tear

20 A 14-year-old female presents to her pediatrician with acute knee pain following a soccer injury. An axial T2-weighted MR image is provided below. Which of the following would predispose a patient to this type of injury?

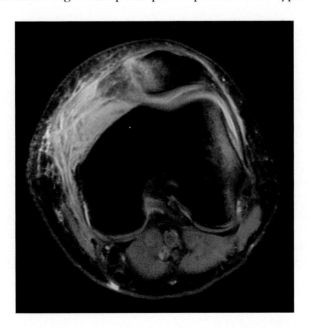

    A. Iliotibial band friction syndrome
    B. Trochlear dysplasia
    C. Patella baja
    D. Vastus medialis muscle hypertrophy
    E. Osgood-Schlatter disease

21 A lateral radiograph of the cervical spine is provided. Which of the following is true regarding the imaged pathology?

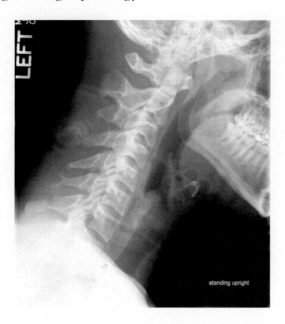

A. Results from abrupt hyperextension.
B. More commonly involves the upper cervical spine.
C. Categorized with the Anderson-D'Alonzo classification system.
D. The injury is mechanically stable.

22 A 44-year-old presents with acute onset of pain and swelling of the calf. Axial and coronal T1- and T2-weighted MR images are provided. What is the most likely diagnosis?

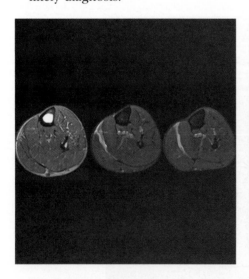
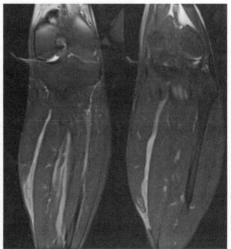

A. Rupture of the medial head of gastrocnemius muscle
B. Rupture of the soleus muscle
C. Dissecting popliteal cyst
D. Rupture of the plantaris tendon
E. Venous varicosity

~ **23** A 30-year-old male presents to the emergency department with shoulder pain. Based on the radiograph below, what is the diagnosis?

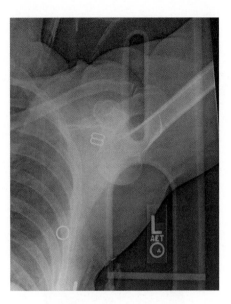

    A. Anterior shoulder dislocation
    B. Luxatio erecta
    C. Hill-Sachs lesion
    D. Posterior shoulder dislocation
    E. Reverse Hill-Sachs lesion

24a In addition to tendinopathy, diabetes, steroid use, and connective tissue disorders, what factor might predispose a patient to suffer the injury pictured in the following MRI?

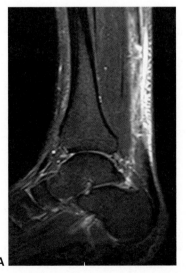
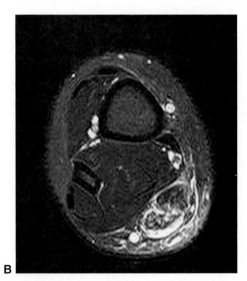

A. Sagittal T2 weighted **B.** Axial T2 weighted

    A. Heavy ethanol use
    B. Human immunodeficiency virus
    C. Recent fluoroquinolone use
    D. Hepatitis C
    E. Recent penicillin use

24b Achilles tendon tears are most likely to occur at which location?

   A. Calcaneal insertion
   B. Myotendinous junction
   C. Midsubstance
   D. Intrasubstance

25 The unopposed action of which tendon causes proximal retraction of the larger fracture fragment in the injury pictured below?

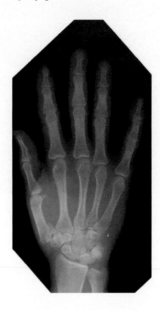

   A. Abductor pollicis
   B. Flexor pollicis longus
   C. Flexor digitorum profundus
   D. Extensor pollicis longus

26 The acetabular labrum is most commonly torn in which quadrant?

   A. Anterior superior
   B. Posterior superior
   C. Anterior inferior
   D. Posterior inferior

27 Which of the following acetabular fractures involves the iliac wing?

   A. Transverse
   B. Posterior wall
   C. T shaped
   D. Both column
   E. Transverse with the posterior wall

28 A 17-year-old male football player is referred to radiology for MR arthrogram of the shoulder. The patient reports a remote anterior subluxation event, and the clinician is concerned that the patient may have an anterior inferior labral tear. Which of the following positions will improve visualization of the anterior inferior labrum?

   A. Flexion, adduction, and internal rotation
   B. Flexion, abduction, and supination
   C. Abduction and external rotation
   D. Arm neutral with internal rotation

29 What is the most common morphology of the meniscal tear depicted below?

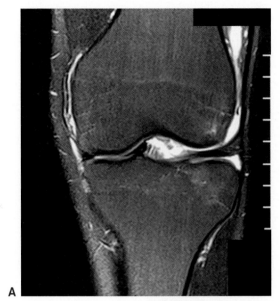
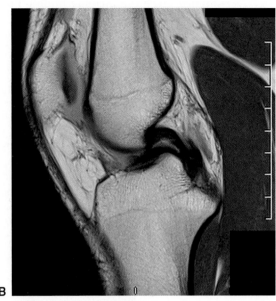

A. Coronal proton density fat saturated **B.** Sagittal proton density

A. Vertical longitudinal
B. Horizontal cleavage
C. Horizontal oblique
D. Radial

30 Complete disruption of which ligament classifies the imaged pathology as a grade III injury as opposed to a grade II injury?

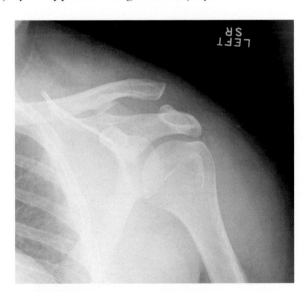

A. Acromioclavicular ligament
B. Coracoclavicular ligament
C. Coracoacromial ligament
D. Coracohumeral ligament

• **31** Which of the following knee structures should be closely evaluated for an injury, given the imaging finding below?

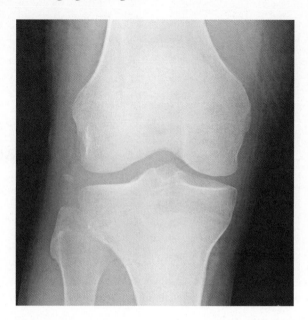

A. Patellar tendon
B. Posterolateral corner
C. Lateral meniscus
D. Proximal tibiofibular joint
E. Popliteal artery

• **32** Additional views of the left shoulder may reveal which finding in the following patient?

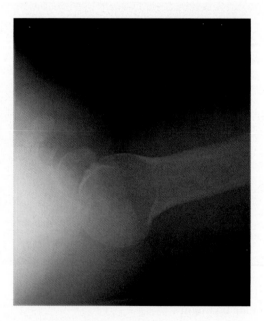

A. Humeral head locked in external rotation on AP images
B. Increased distance between the articular cortex of the humeral head and glenoid rim
C. Impaction fracture of the posterolateral humeral head
D. Fracture of the anteroinferior glenoid

33 In the injury pictured, entrapment of the ulnar collateral ligament superficial to what structure may result in a Stener lesion, resulting in the need for surgical management?

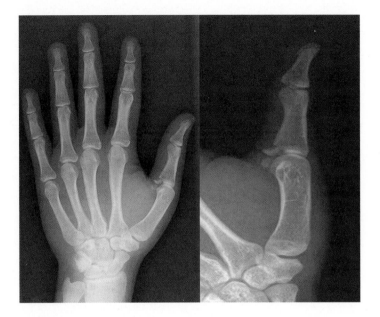

   A. Adductor aponeurosis
   B. Radial collateral ligament
   C. Extensor hood
   D. Flexor pollicis longus

34 A patient complains of persistent knee pain following repeated hyperextension injuries experienced while playing basketball 2 months prior. Sagittal proton density and proton density fat-saturated images through the intercondylar notch are provided. Imaging findings are classic for which of the following injuries?

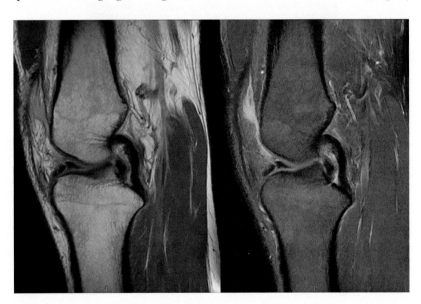

   A. Bucket handle tear of the lateral meniscus
   B. Radial tear of the medial meniscus
   C. Bucket handle tear of the medial meniscus
   D. Partial-thickness tear of the posterior cruciate ligament

` **35** A 19-year-old female runner presents with acutely worsening hip pain. What grade stress injury/stress fracture is depicted in the coronal T2-weighted fat-saturated MR image below?

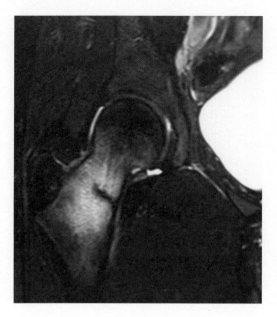

A. Grade 0
B. Grade 1
C. Grade 2
D. Grade 3
E. Grade 4

36 If emergent surgical management of the imaged injury is not performed, what additional radiologic study should be performed next?

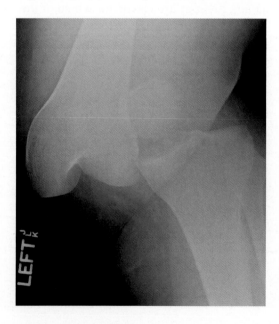

A. MRI of the knee without contrast
B. MRI of the knee with contrast
C. CT angiography of the lower extremity
D. Noncontrast CT of the lower extremity

37a A frontal ankle radiograph is provided. Which modality is best suited to estimate the stability of this lesion?

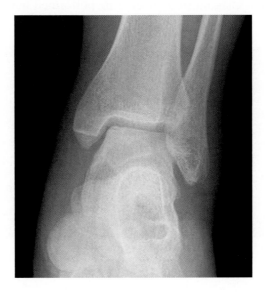

A. CT
B. Ultrasound
C. Tc-99m bone scan
D. MRI

37b MRI findings that would indicate that the above osteochondral lesion is unstable would include

A. fluid signal interface with the donor bone.
B. granulation tissue interface with the donor bone.
C. absence of adjacent cyst-like change.
D. overlying cartilage fissure.

38 What is the prevailing mechanism responsible for the injury pictured below?

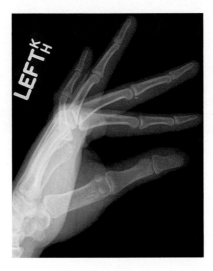

A. Hyperextension of the proximal interphalangeal joint
B. Hyperflexion of the proximal interphalangeal joint
C. Avulsion of the flexor digitorum profundus tendon
D. Avulsion of the central slip of the extensor digitorum tendon

39 After a fall on an outstretched hand, a patient complains of elbow pain. Radiographs were obtained in the emergency department. Based on the radiographs, what imaging study should be performed next in the emergent setting?

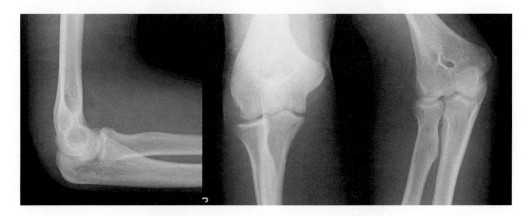

A. MRI
B. CT
C. Stress radiographs
D. Ultrasound

40 An axial proton density fat-saturated MR image of the upper leg is provided. Injury to what structure could result in the findings below?

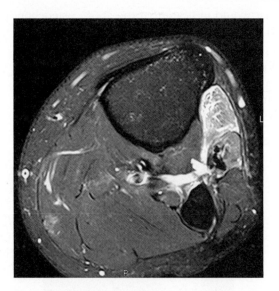

A. Tibial nerve
B. Peroneal nerve
C. Popliteal nerve
D. Sciatic nerve

41 Which of the following is the first radiographic manifestation of fracture healing?

A. Callus formation about the fracture site
B. Filling in of callus between the fracture fragments
C. Widening of the fracture line with blurring of fracture margins
D. Demineralization of the adjacent bone around the fracture

42 An oblique radiograph of the left foot is provided. Avulsion of what structure could produce these findings?

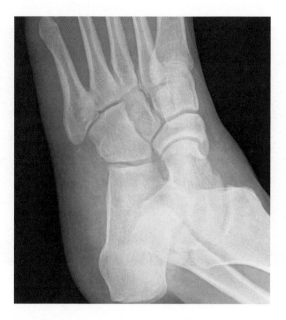

A. Peroneus longus
B. Abductor digiti minimi
C. Lateral plantar aponeurosis
D. Peroneal retinaculum

43a Coronal T2-weighted fat-saturated and sagittal T1-weighted MR images of the shoulder are provided. Which of the following best describes the imaging findings?

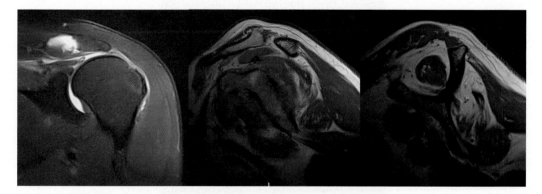

A. Full-thickness rotator cuff tear with fatty atrophy of the infraspinatus
B. Full-thickness rotator cuff tear with fatty atrophy of the teres minor
C. Full-thickness rotator cuff tear with fatty atrophy of the subscapularis
D. Full-thickness rotator cuff tear with fatty atrophy of the deltoid

43b Rotator cuff tears most commonly involve which tendon?

A. Supraspinatus
B. Subscapularis
C. Infraspinatus
D. Teres minor

44 The 3D CT images below demonstrate the most common mechanism for ankle fracture. What is the mechanism, according to the Lauge-Hansen classification system?

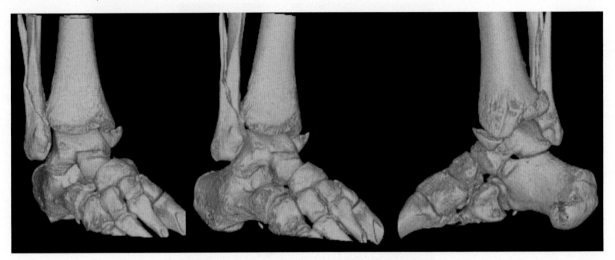

    A. Supination adduction
    B. Supination external rotation
    C. Pronation external rotation
    D. Pronation abduction

45 A single axial CT image of the cervical spine is provided. The imaging findings are consistent with what unstable cervical spine injury?

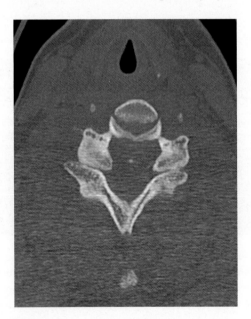

    A. Flexion teardrop fracture
    B. Bilateral interfacetal dislocation
    C. Unilateral perched facet
    D. Cervical burst fracture

‹ **46** The Pellegrini-Stieda lesion indicates injury to which structure?

   A. ACL
   B. PCL
   C. LCL
   D. MCL

ˀ **47a** An 18-year-old hockey player complains of pain after sustaining an injury. Where is the injury?

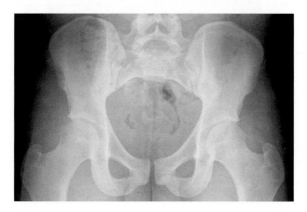

   A. Right hip
   B. Left hip
   C. Sacrum
   D. Pubic symphysis
   E. Soft tissues

47b Based on the MR images, what is the most likely mechanism of injury?

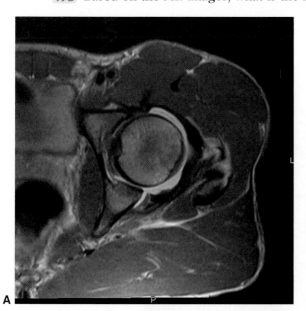
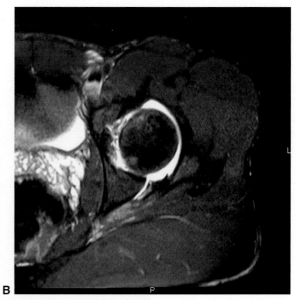

A. Axial proton density **B.** Axial T2 weighted fat saturated

   A. Anterior dislocation
   B. Posterior dislocation
   C. Internal rotation
   D. External rotation

48 A 47-year-old male suffered high-voltage electrical burn injuries to his feet bilaterally when a metallic tent pole he was assembling contacted a power line. Which of the following is true regarding the imaging findings associated with musculoskeletal thermal trauma?

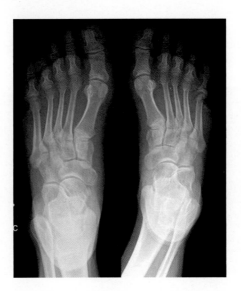

A. Frostbite-related acroosteolysis most commonly involves the thumb.

B. The physes of skeletally immature patients are relatively resistant to thermal trauma.

C. Resulting muscular fatty atrophy will manifest as areas of T1 prolongation on MRI.

D. Imaging findings may include dystrophic calcification or heterotopic ossification.

49 The combination of injuries seen on the provided radiographs of the right elbow and wrist has been named

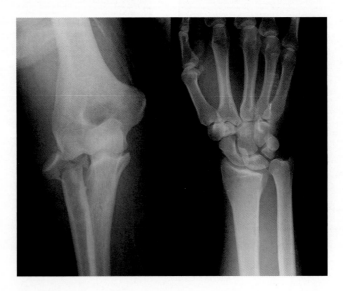

A. Essex-Lopresti fracture.

B. Monteggia fracture.

C. Galeazzi fracture.

D. nightstick fracture.

50 A fracture in which region of the scaphoid is most susceptible to developing avascular necrosis?

    A. Proximal pole
    B. Waist
    C. Distal pole
    D. Tubercle

51a A frontal radiograph of the knee is provided. This finding has a >90% association with injury to what structure?

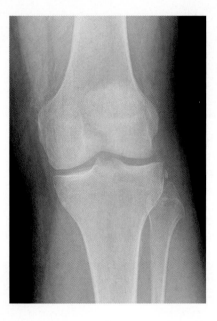

    A. Biceps femoris tendon
    B. Popliteus tendon
    C. Anterior cruciate ligament
    D. Posterior cruciate ligament
    E. Lateral meniscus

51b A mirror image injury to that seen in 51a can also occur, with avulsion of the tibial attachment of the capsular portion of the deep medial collateral ligament. This so-called reverse Segond fracture has a high association with injury to what structure?

    A. Semimembranosus tendon
    B. Medial head of gastrocnemius
    C. Anterior cruciate ligament
    D. Posterior cruciate ligament
    E. Lateral meniscus

52 Which of the following proximal femoral fractures is most susceptible to avascular necrosis?

    A. Intertrochanteric
    B. Subtrochanteric
    C. Trochanteric
    D. Subcapital

53 A 45-year-old man complains of shoulder pain after a fall. Based on the images below, what is the best diagnosis?

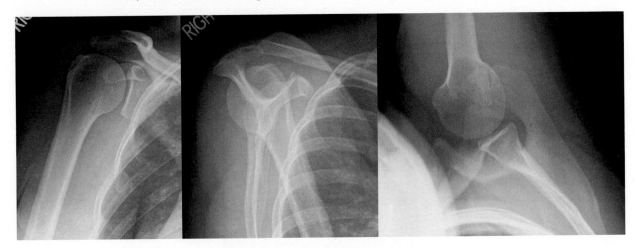

    A. Sequela of anterior dislocation
    B. Sequela of posterior dislocation
    C. Nondisplaced fracture
    D. Normal variant

54 A 22-year-old college football player experiences acute groin pain after an injury. From the single provided image below, what is the diagnosis?

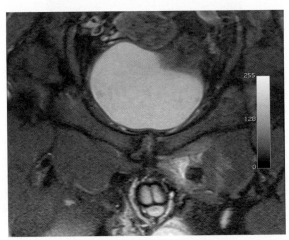

Axial oblique T2 weighted fat saturated

    A. Acute right-sided athletic pubalgia
    B. Acute left-sided athletic pubalgia
    C. Right-sided inguinal hernia
    D. Left-sided inguinal hernia
    E. Stress fracture of the pubis

55 Which of the following nerves is most likely entrapped in the clinical setting of forearm pain with weakness of the extensors and preserved sensation?

    A. Median nerve
    B. Radial nerve
    C. Ulnar nerve
    D. Anterior interosseous nerve
    E. Posterior interosseous nerve

56 A 19-year-old basketball player presents with chronic anterior knee pain. Based on the imaging findings below, which clinical entity is demonstrated?

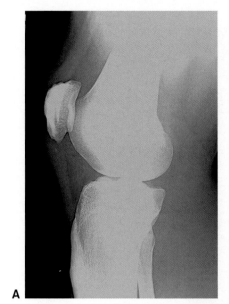 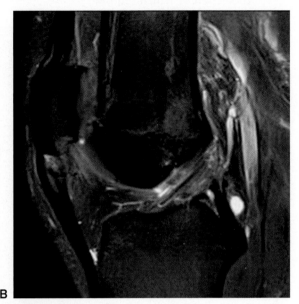

A. Lateral radiograph **B.** Sagittal proton density fat saturated

A. Runner's knee
B. Jumper's knee
C. Hoffa syndrome
D. Tennis leg

57 A 19-year-old male presents with a radial side mass and remote history of trauma to the elbow. Radiographs reveal only soft tissue swelling. The ultrasound images below depict what type of foreign body?

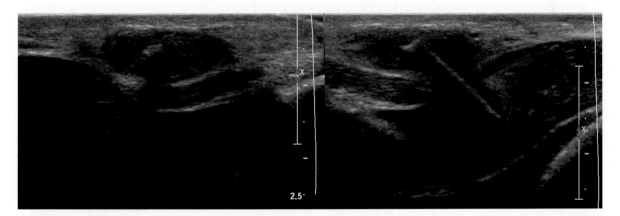

A. Metal
B. Stone
C. Wood
D. Glass

58 The patient suffered an injury resulting in forceful hyperflexion of the distal phalanx of the small finger. Retraction of the avulsed fragment is the result of the action of which tendon?

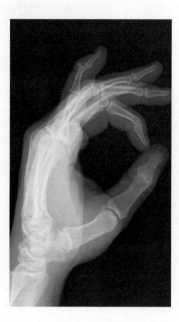

A. Extensor digiti minimi
B. Flexor digitorum superficialis
C. Flexor digitorum profundus
D. Extensor carpi ulnaris
E. Extensor indicis

59a Axial T2-weighted fat-saturated MR images of the glenohumeral joint and midhumerus are provided. The images depict what abnormality?

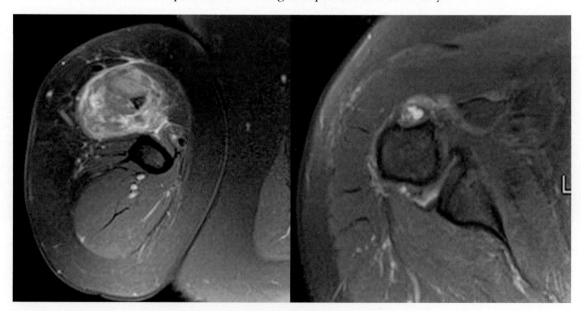

A. Long head of biceps tendon rupture
B. Pectoralis major tendon rupture
C. Short head of biceps tendon rupture
D. Coracobrachialis tendon rupture

59b Long head of biceps tendon rupture most commonly occurs in what location?

    A. Distal radial attachment
    B. Proximal intra-articular portion
    C. Proximal intertubercular portion
    D. Lacertus fibrosis

60 Based on the findings below, what was the most likely mechanism of injury?

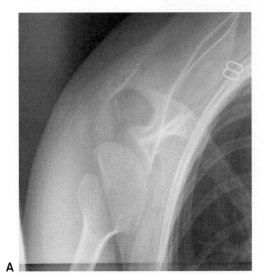 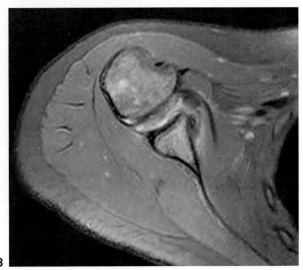

A. Axillary radiograph **B.** Axial proton density fat saturated

    A. Direct anterior impaction
    B. Anterior dislocation
    C. Posterior dislocation
    D. Contrecoup injury

61 A patient presents to the emergency department following an MVC. Which of the following is true regarding the imaged fracture complication?

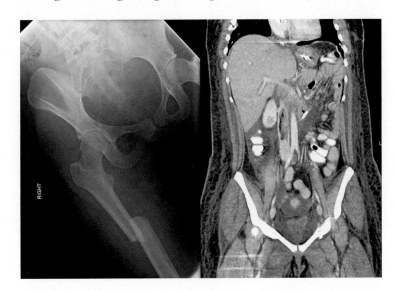

    A. Most commonly occurs following lumbar spine burst fractures.
    B. Can be associated with petechial rash, hypoxia, and altered mental status.
    C. CT angiography is usually highly specific for the diagnosis of this entity.
    D. VQ scan usually shows large central segmental mismatched perfusion defects.

62 A collegiate football player suffered a foot injury while practicing. Radiographs were interpreted as normal, and an MRI was subsequently performed. The requisition states, "concern for Lisfranc injury." What is the actual diagnosis?

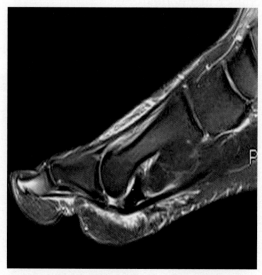

Sagittal T2 weighted fat saturated

A. Flexor hallucis longus tendon tear
B. Abductor hallucis tendon tear
C. Plantar plate injury
D. Intersesamoid ligament tear

63 A 25-year-old runner complains of lateral knee pain that is worse with activity. Radiographs were performed and were interpreted as normal. Two images from an MR are provided below. What is the correct diagnosis?

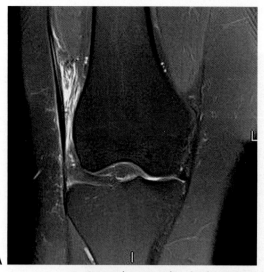 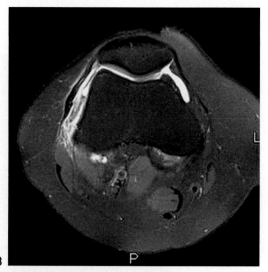

A. Coronal proton density fat saturated **B.** Axial proton density fat saturated

A. Iliotibial band tear
B. Iliotibial band syndrome
C. Vastus lateralis muscle tear
D. Bone contusion
E. Fibular collateral ligament tear

64 Sublabral foramen and Buford complex, anatomic variants of the glenoid labrum, occur in which quadrant of the labrum?

    A. Posteroinferior
    B. Posterosuperior
    C. Anteroinferior
    D. Anterosuperior

65 A 25-year-old patient complains of wrist pain and swelling after a fall. Three radiographs of the wrist are provided. What is the most likely diagnosis?

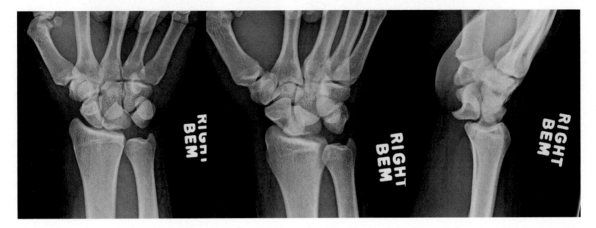

    A. Perilunate dislocation
    B. Lunate dislocation
    C. Transscaphoid perilunate dislocation
    D. Scaphocapitate fracture dislocation

66 3D CT images of the glenoid are provided. What imaging criterion is commonly used as a cutoff to determine the need for surgical fixation or bone grafting as a means of restoring stability?

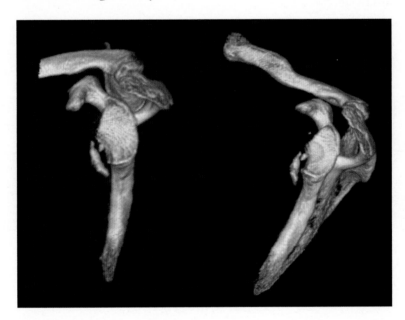

    A. 10% glenoid surface bone loss
    B. 25% glenoid surface bone loss
    C. 50% glenoid surface bone loss
    D. 75 % glenoid surface bone loss

67 A patient presents with inability to extend the knee following an injury. Which of the following is true regarding the imaged pathology?

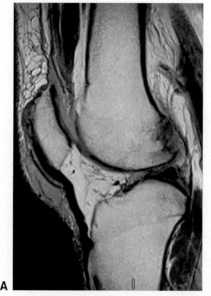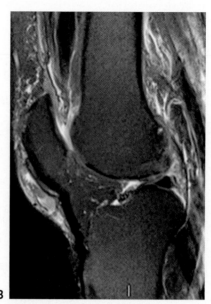

A. Sagittal proton density **B.** Sagittal proton density fat saturated

A. May be associated with patella alta.
B. Partial-thickness injuries most commonly involve the vastus medialis.
C. Both partial- and full-thickness tears are usually managed conservatively.
D. May be associated with avulsion fractures of the superior patella.

68a T1-weighted and T2-weighted fat-saturated MR images of the ankle are provided, as well as a lateral radiograph. Which term correctly describes osseous excrescences at the calcaneal insertion of the Achilles tendon and the plantar fascia?

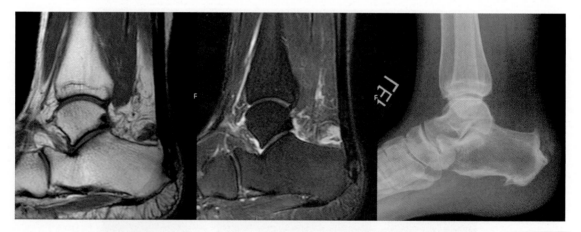

A. Osteophyte
B. Periostitis
C. Enthesophyte
D. Osteochondrosis

68b The provided images suggest what diagnosis?

   A. Sever disease with retrocalcaneal bursitis
   B. Calcaneal stress fracture with retrocalcaneal bursitis
   C. Haglund deformity with retrocalcaneal bursitis
   D. Plantar fasciitis with retrocalcaneal bursitis

69a A 20-year-old collegiate athlete presented for imaging following an injury suffered during a football game. Sagittal and axial T2-weighted fat-saturated MR images demonstrate injury to the origin of what structure?

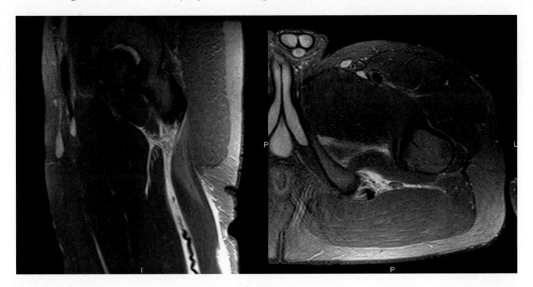

   A. Gluteus medius tendon
   B. Adductor longus tendon
   C. Hamstring muscle complex tendons
   D. Gluteus maximus tendon
   E. Iliopsoas tendon

69b What specific hamstring muscle complex tendon injury is depicted in the images above?

   A. Biceps femoris
   B. Semimembranosus
   C. Semitendinosus
   D. Sartorius

70 Which of the following structures represents boundaries or contents of the rotator interval of the shoulder?

   A. Short head of the biceps tendon
   B. Middle glenohumeral ligament
   C. Coracoclavicular ligament
   D. Superior glenohumeral ligament
   E. Coracoacromial ligament
   F. Inferior glenohumeral ligament

71   A 45-year-old female complains of elbow pain. Based on the T2-weighted fat-saturated MR images, which choice below correctly localizes the abnormality?

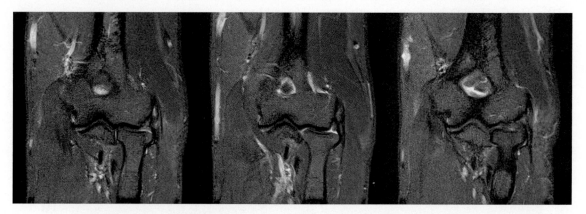

  A. Common extensor origin
  B. Common flexor origin
  C. Ulnar collateral ligament
  D. Radial collateral ligament

72   A 16-year-old high school wrestler presents with a painful anterior knee mass. A lateral knee radiograph is provided, as well as an axial T2-weighted fat-saturated and axial T1-weighted fat-saturated postcontrast MR image. Which of the following correctly identifies the site of the abnormality?

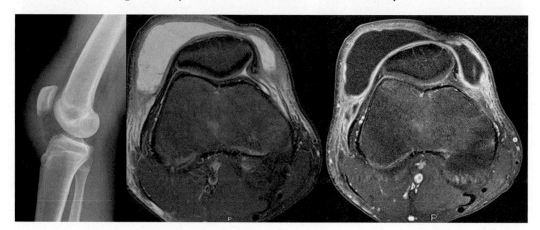

  A. Suprapatellar bursa
  B. Deep infrapatellar bursa
  C. Pes anserine bursa
  D. Prepatellar bursa
  E. Superficial infrapatellar bursa

73 Axial and coronal T2-weighted fat-saturated MR images of a football player who sustained an ankle injury are shown below. What is the diagnosis?

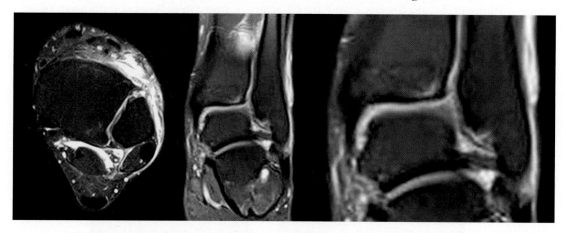

A. Anterior talofibular ligament tear
B. Posterior talofibular ligament tear
C. Anteroinferior tibiofibular ligament tear
D. Posteroinferior tibiofibular ligament tear
E. Calcaneofibular ligament tear

74 The imaged pathology most commonly occurs at what specific site in the knee in adolescent patients?

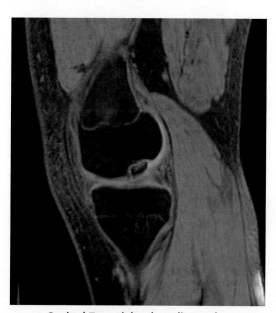

Sagittal T2-weighted gradient echo

A. Lateral weight-bearing aspect of the medial femoral condyle
B. Medial weight-bearing aspect of the medial femoral condyle
C. Lateral weight-bearing aspect of the lateral femoral condyle
D. Medial weight-bearing aspect of the lateral femoral condyle

75 A 50-year-old complains of persistent pain following a left wrist injury. The initial radiographs of the wrist at the time of injury, 6-week follow-up radiograph, and 6-week follow-up CT scan are presented. What complication of the injury is shown in the 6-week follow-up radiograph and CT scan?

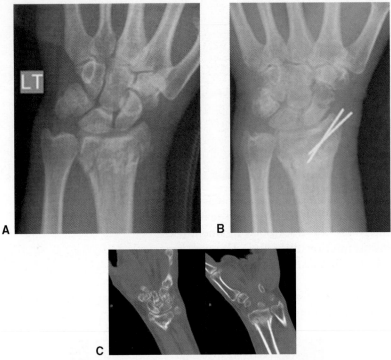

A. Initial radiograph **B.** 6-week follow-up radiograph **C.** 6-week follow-up CT

A. Reflex sympathetic dystrophy
B. Fracture nonunion
C. Hardware failure
D. Avascular necrosis

76a PA and lateral radiographs of the wrist are obtained after a patient suffers a fall on an outstretched hand. What is the diagnosis?

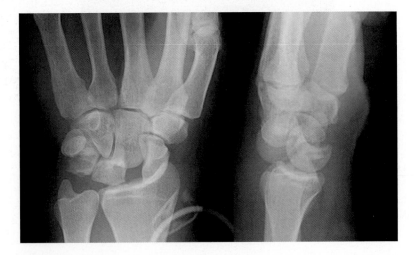

A. Perilunate dislocation
B. Scapholunate dissociation
C. Lunate dislocation
D. Midcarpal dislocation

76b Lesser arch injuries of the wrist progress through the following joint spaces in a predictable pattern. Which of the following choices correctly orders the injury progression, from least to greatest severity?

A. Scapholunate; lunotriquetral; lunocapitate
B. Lunotriquetral; lunocapitate; scapholunate
C. Scapholunate; lunocapitate; lunotriquetral
D. Lunocapitate; lunotriquetral; scapholunate

77 A high school sprinter complains of several weeks of ankle pain and is referred for MR imaging. Based on the images below, what is the most appropriate management of this patient?

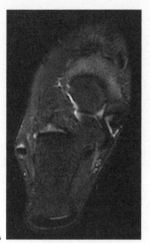 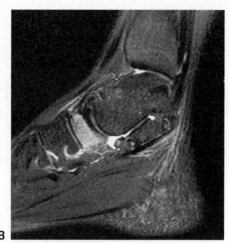

A. Axial T2 weighted fat saturated **B.** Coronal T2 weighted fat saturated

A. External fixation
B. Prophylactic internal fixation
C. Immobilization and non–weight bearing
D. No treatment necessary, return to sprinting

78 A 61-year-old male was involved in a farming accident. Bedside probing of the wound demonstrates extensive associated soft tissue injury. Initial management of the fracture will likely consist of which of the following?

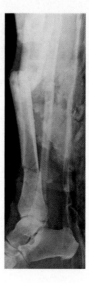

A. Intramedullary nail
B. External fixation
C. Plate fixation
D. Interfragmentary screws

79   A 22-year-old college student presents with knee pain with extension after anterior cruciate ligament reconstruction. The referring physician is concerned for a tear of the graft. What is the diagnosis?

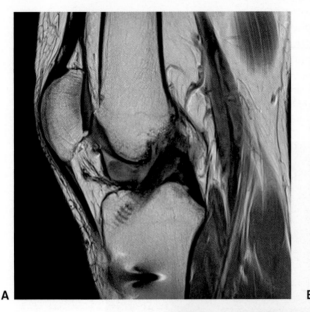

A

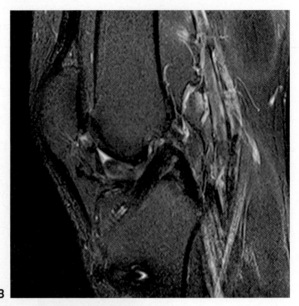

B

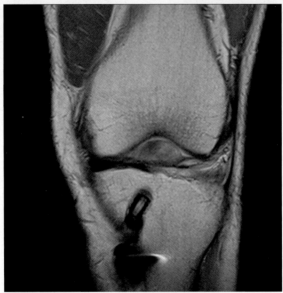

C

A. Sagittal proton density **B.** Sagittal proton density fat saturated **C.** Coronal T1 weighted

    A. Anterior cruciate graft tear
    B. Posterior cruciate ligament tear
    C. Meniscus tear
    D. Arthrofibrosis

80 Two sequential coronal T1-weighted fat-saturated images from an elbow
arthrogram are provided. What is the prevailing mechanism responsible for the
injury depicted?

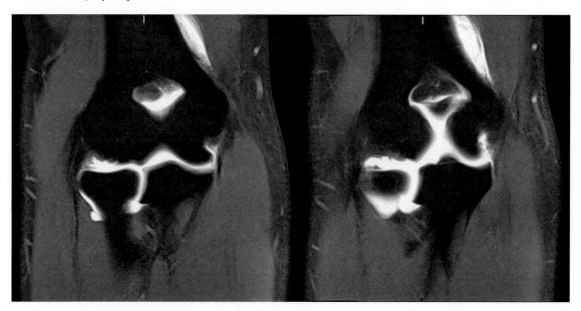

A. Repetitive excessive varus stress
B. Hyperextension injury
C. Distraction injury
D. Repetitive excessive valgus stress

ANSWERS AND EXPLANATIONS

1 **Answer A.** Pivot shift injury occurs when there is a valgus load applied to the knee while the knee is in various states of flexion. The knee flexion is combined with external rotation of the tibia or internal rotation of the femur. This injury is commonly seen in American football players. The resultant bone contusions are located at the lateral femoral condyle and posterolateral margin of the tibial plateau. The contusions occur after the ACL tears and allow anterior subluxation of the tibia with respect to the femur.

Reference: Sanders TG, Medynski MA, Feller JF, et al. Bone contusion patterns of the knee at MR imaging: footprint of the mechanism of injury. *Radiographics.* 2000;20:S135–S151.

2 **Answer E.** The extensor tendons are the dorsal tendons of the wrist and are superficial to the capsule of the wrist. They extend to insert on the carpal bones and phalanges. There are six extensor compartments, which are numbered from the radial to ulnar direction. The compartments are best delineated on axial sequences. Compartment I is composed of the abductor pollicis longus and extensor pollicis brevis tendons and is located along the lateral border of the radius. Compartment II contains the extensor carpi radialis longus and extensor carpi radialis brevis tendons. Compartment II rests along the dorsal and lateral aspect of the radius. Compartment III includes the extensor pollicis longus tendon. Compartment IV is composed of the extensor digitorum and extensor indicis tendons with a shared tendon sheath. The extensor digiti minimi tendon is in Compartment V. Compartment VI contains the extensor carpi ulnaris. Compartments II and III are separated by Lister tubercle, a bony ridge at the dorsal radius.

Reference: Stein JM, Cook TS, Simonson S, et al. Normal and variant anatomy of the wrist and hand on MR imaging. *Magn Reson Imaging Clin N Am* 2011;19:595–608.

3 **Answer B.** The provided radiographs demonstrate medial clear space widening and posterior malleolar irregularity. There is no fibular fracture on the provided images. The medial clear space widening indicates deltoid ligament injury. With deltoid ligament injury and a posterior malleolar fracture, the mechanism of injury is pronation–lateral rotation by the Lauge-Hansen classification. A radiograph of the tibia/fibula should be performed with these findings as the posterior malleolar fracture classifies this injury as stage IV. If there is no posterior malleolus fracture, the injury is pronation–lateral rotation stage III. The fibular fracture in pronation–lateral rotation injuries typically occurs anywhere from 6 cm proximal to the tibial plafond to the fibular neck.

Reference: Arimoto HK, Forrester DM. Classification of ankle fractures: an algorithm. *AJR Am J Roentgenol.* 1980;135:1057–1063.

4a **Answer D.** Images show a T2-weighted, hyperintense cystic mass within the spinoglenoid notch, without extension into the suprascapular notch. The suprascapular notch is noted superior to the spine of the scapula within the suprascapular fossa and is covered by the superior transverse scapular ligament. From the suprascapular fossa, the nerve continues inferiorly and laterally to the spinoglenoid notch, through which it enters the infraspinous fossa. The spinoglenoid notch may be covered by the spinoglenoid ligament in up to 80% of individuals. The quadrilateral space is bounded inferiorly by the teres major, superiorly by the teres minor, laterally by the humeral neck, and medially by the long head of triceps. The rotator interval is the space bounded by the cranial subscapularis and anterior supraspinatus and contains the superior glenohumeral ligament, coracohumeral ligament, and long head of the biceps tendon.

Reference: Sonin A, Manaster BJ, Andrews CL, et al. *Diagnostic Imaging: Musculoskeletal: Trauma*. Manitoba, Canada: Amirsys; 2010:2:172–173.

4b **Answer C.** A paralabral cyst in the spinoglenoid notch can impinge upon the suprascapular nerve and result in denervation of the infraspinatus muscle. When the mass extends into the suprascapular notch, branches to both the supraspinatus and infraspinatus muscles may be compressed. Masses or fibrous bands in the quadrilateral space may compress the axillary nerve, resulting in denervation of the teres minor and deltoid. Masses in the rotator interval do not compress the suprascapular or axillary nerve.

Reference: Sonin A, Manaster BJ, Andrews CL, et al. *Diagnostic Imaging: Musculoskeletal: Trauma*. Manitoba, Canada: Amirsys; 2010:2:172–173.

5 **Answer C.** The coronal T1-weighted image shows replacement of the expected fatty marrow signal within the lunate by diffuse T1 hypointensity. The lunate demonstrates an abnormal configuration with flattening. These findings are compatible with lunate osteonecrosis, also called Kienböck disease. After AVN of the proximal pole of the scaphoid, the lunate is the most likely carpal bone to undergo osteonecrosis. The injury results from damage to the tenuous blood supply to the bone, usually from chronic repetitive microtrauma such as that occurs in manual laborers. Ulnar negative variance is often associated with this pathology, due to altered force distribution across the lunate. Ulnar positive variance can be associated with ulnolunate abutment syndrome, resulting in tears of the triangular fibrocartilage and ulnolunate degenerative arthrosis. Distal radioulnar impingement refers to impingement of an abnormally shortened distal ulna against the radius proximal to the sigmoid notch.

Reference: Morrison WB, Sanders TG. *Problem Solving in Musculoskeletal Imaging*. Philadelphia, PA: Mosby; 2008:464–467.

6 **Answer A.** Heterotopic ossification is formation of bone and cartilage in soft tissue. It is also referred to as myositis ossificans and is a benign entity. Initially, it manifests as a soft tissue mass. Approximately 4 weeks after the insult, osteoid begins to form and there may be periosteal reaction. The bone continues to mature, and after 6 months, cortical bone is present peripherally. There may be internal trabecula. Patients often present with pain, tenderness, swelling, and a palpable mass. Predisposing factors include trauma, surgery, burns, and neurologic insults including spinal cord injury. Patients with a history of hip arthroplasty are at risk for local heterotopic ossification. Of the other answer choices, tumoral calcinosis is also separate from the bone, but the mass is calcified and not ossified. Parosteal osteosarcoma is a low-grade sarcoma that occurs on the surface of bones. An osteochondroma contains mature bone similar to heterotopic ossification, but there is corticomedullary continuity between the normal bone and the osteochondroma. Osteochondromas usually arise from the metaphysis.

Reference: Manaster BJ, Roberts CC, Petersilge CA, et al. *Diagnostic Imaging: Musculoskeletal: Non-Traumatic Disease*. Manitoba, Canada: Amirsys; 2010:3:262–267.

7a **Answer C.** Images show edema along the expected course of the distal biceps tendon, with absence of the tendon at its distal attachment onto the radial tuberosity. While the axial images alone could potentially be confused with a tear of the brachialis tendon (so-called climber elbow), the sagittal images clearly demonstrate an intact brachialis muscle and tendon. Bicipitoradial bursitis may be seen in association with biceps tendon tears; however, in bursitis alone, the tendon would remain intact. Cephalic vein thrombosis would present as the absence of a flow void in the expected location of the cephalic vein.

References: Morrison WB, Sanders TG. *Problem Solving in Musculoskeletal Imaging.* Philadelphia, PA: Mosby; 2008:412.
Sonin A, Manaster BJ, Andrews CL, et al. *Diagnostic Imaging: Musculoskeletal: Trauma.* Manitoba, Canada: Amirsys; 2010:3:74–79.

7b Answer C. Distal biceps tendon rupture is usually evident clinically. The role of MR imaging is to differentiate partial from complete disruption and to determine the extent of retraction. An intact lacertus fibrosus (bicipital aponeurosis) may prevent proximal retraction of the biceps tendon even if a complete tear has occurred.

References: Morrison WB, Sanders TG. *Problem Solving in Musculoskeletal Imaging.* Philadelphia, PA: Mosby; 2008:412.
Sonin A, Manaster BJ, Andrews CL, et al. *Diagnostic Imaging: Musculoskeletal: Trauma.* Manitoba, Canada: Amirsys; 2010:3:74–79.

8 Answer E. The image depicts avulsion of the anterior superior iliac spine, the attachment site of the sartorius. This injury can commonly be seen in kicking athletes and can be the result of a single episode of forceful contraction or repetitive overuse. Other pelvic and hip avulsion injuries include anterior inferior iliac spine (rectus femoris), ischial tuberosity (semimembranosus and semitendinosus), greater trochanter (gluteus medius), and lesser trochanter (iliopsoas). Tear or detachment of the rectus abdominis aponeurosis from the anteroinferior pubic symphysis is one of the several causes of athletic pubalgia, formerly referred to as a sports hernia. A classic teaching is that, in the adult patient, avulsion of the iliopsoas from the lesser trochanter should raise concern for a pathologic fracture.

Reference: Sanders TG, Zlatkin MB. Avulsion injuries of the pelvis. *Semin Musculoskelet Radiol.* 2008;12:42–53.

9 Answer B. Galeazzi fracture consists of a radial shaft fracture (usually mid- to distal shaft) with an associated distal radioulnar joint dislocation. The Essex-Lopresti fracture is a radial head fracture with dislocation of the distal radioulnar joint. The radial head fracture is usually comminuted. Monteggia fracture/dislocation is an anterior dislocation of the radial head with a fracture of the proximal third of the ulna. Barton fracture is an intra-articular fracture of the distal radius with subluxation or dislocation of the wrist. The fracture may be volar or dorsal. The Smith fracture is also known as the reverse Colles fracture where there is a distal radius fracture without intra-articular extension. There is volar displacement of the distal fracture fragment in the Smith fracture.

References: Hunter TB, Peltier LF, Lund PJ. Radiologic history exhibit. Musculoskeletal eponyms: who are those guys? *Radiographics.* 2000;20:819–836.
Lee P, Hunter TB, Taljanovic M. Musculoskeletal colloquialisms: how did we come up with these names? *Radiographics.* 2004;24:1009–1027.

10 Answer D. Shoulder dislocations are most commonly anterior, referring to the location of the humeral head relative to the glenoid fossa. Posterior dislocations are rare, accounting for 2% of shoulder dislocations. Most posterior dislocations can be classified as subacromial and are fixed with the humeral head trapped posterior to the glenoid. There is commonly an associated humeral head fracture. Posterior dislocation is commonly the result of violent muscle contractions in the setting of seizures. The shoulder can also posteriorly dislocate as a result of electric shock or a direct anterior blow to the shoulder. Posterior dislocation can be subtle radiographically. On frontal radiographs of the shoulder, it may manifest as severe internal rotation of the humeral head resembling a light bulb or the rim sign. In the rim sign, there is increased distance between the glenoid and articular surface of the humeral head. Posterior dislocation can also manifest as the trough line sign on frontal radiographs. When the humeral head posteriorly dislocates, it impacts the posterior glenoid. The impaction at the medial humeral head has a linear configuration and is called the trough line sign. This fracture is sometimes referred to as the reverse Hill-Sachs fracture.

References: Gor DM. The trough line sign. *Radiology.* 2002;224:485–486.
Pope TL, Harris JH. *Harris and Harris' the Radiology of Emergency Medicine.* 5th ed. Philadelphia, PA: Lippincott Williams & Wilkins; 2013:319–320, 326–328.

11 **Answer C.** The Lisfranc ligament spans the medial cuneiform-second metatarsal base. This structure is crucial to stabilization of the midfoot and longitudinal arch. The radiographic findings include widening of the space between the first and second metatarsals, abnormal tarsal–metatarsal alignment, and dorsal migration of the metatarsal bases. Injuries are commonly classified as homolateral or divergent based upon the direction of dislocation of the first metatarsal with respect to that of the metatarsals two through five. In Lisfranc injuries, the ligament may avulse from the second metatarsal or medial cuneiform or may tear within its substance without associated fracture.

References: Morrison WB, Sanders TG. *Problem Solving in Musculoskeletal Imaging.* Philadelphia, PA: Mosby; 2008:702–705.
Pope TL, Harris JH. *Harris and Harris' the Radiology of Emergency Medicine.* 5th ed. Philadelphia, PA: Lippincott Williams & Wilkins; 2013:962–965.

12 **Answer B.** A cross-table lateral view of the knee shows a layered joint effusion, with the more lucent-nondependent layer representing lipid. The presence of both blood and fat within the joint space is highly specific for an intra-articular fracture, with the fat layer representing that which has leaked into the joint from the marrow cavity. Further imaging should be performed to identify the fracture, if not seen radiographically.

Reference: Pope TL, Harris JH. *Harris and Harris' the Radiology of Emergency Medicine.* 5th ed. Philadelphia, PA: Lippincott Williams & Wilkins; 2013:876–877.

13 **Answer A.** A Jones fracture is defined as a transverse fracture of the fifth metatarsal at the junction of the proximal metaphysis and diaphysis, without extension distal to the level of the fourth and fifth intermetatarsal articulations. A tuberosity avulsion fracture occurs proximal to a Jones fracture and results from avulsion of the peroneus brevis tendon and plantar aponeurosis. The avulsion fracture is the most common proximal fifth metatarsal fracture. A fifth metatarsal proximal diaphyseal stress fracture occurs distal to a Jones fracture and normally is seen within the proximal 1.5 cm of the fifth metatarsal diaphysis. Fifth metatarsal stress fractures are the least common proximal fifth metatarsal fractures.

Reference: Theodorou DJ, Theodorou SJ, Kakitsubata Y, et al. Fractures of proximal portion of fifth metatarsal bone: anatomic and imaging evidence of a pathogenesis of avulsion of the plantar aponeurosis and the short peroneal muscle tendon. *Radiology.* 2003;226:857–865.

14 **Answer E.** MR images of the wrist demonstrate fluid within the tendon sheaths of the first extensor compartment and adjacent soft tissue inflammatory changes, findings compatible with de Quervain tenosynovitis. Tenosynovitis involving the abductor pollicis longus and extensor pollicis brevis tendons in this location produces radial wrist pain and swelling. De Quervain tenosynovitis may result from a variety of activities that produce repetitive microtrauma, such as rowing, golfing, or racquet sports. De Quervain tenosynovitis is also referred to as baby wrist overuse syndrome. First extensor compartment inflammation is commonly seen in mothers of newborns due to repeated extension or flexion of the wrist with abduction of the thumb against resistance. This diagnosis can also be made via wrist ultrasound, which would demonstrate fluid within the tendon sheaths of the first extensor compartment and focal increased vascularity.

Reference: Anderson SE, Steinbach LS, De Monaco D, et al. "Baby wrist": MRI of an overuse syndrome in mothers. *AJR Am J Roentgenol.* 2004;182:719–724.

15 Answer C.   The anterior "kissing contusion" pattern is seen when the anterior aspect of the tibial plateau contacts the anterior aspect of the femoral condyle. Hyperextension can be direct, with force applied to the anterior tibia, or indirect such as in forceful kicking.

Reference: Sanders TG, Medynski MA, Feller JF, et al. Bone contusion patterns of the knee at MR imaging: footprint of the mechanism of injury. *Radiographics.* 2000;20:S135–S151.

16 Answer B.   The radiographic images demonstrate widening of the acromioclavicular joint. There is distal clavicle resorption as evidenced by the irregularity of the distal clavicle best seen on the axillary view. There are several bone fragments along the undersurface of the distal clavicle that may be related to prior coracoclavicular ligament injury. Unilateral distal clavicular osteolysis is usually posttraumatic. Osteomyelitis and metastatic disease or myeloma can also cause unilateral distal clavicular osteolysis. Bilateral distal clavicular osteolysis is more likely the result of systemic conditions including hyperparathyroidism, rheumatoid arthritis, and scleroderma. Posttraumatic osteolysis of the distal clavicle occurs after repetitive microtrauma or acute acromioclavicular joint trauma. Classically, distal clavicular osteolysis is seen in weight lifters as a result of chronic stress at the acromioclavicular joint. Early radiographic findings of distal clavicular osteolysis include swelling of the acromioclavicular joint, joint space widening, distal clavicle demineralization, and loss of the distal clavicle cortex. Over time, the cortical margin can reconstitute. Distal clavicle subchondral cysts are a chronic finding.

Reference: Morrison WB, Sanders TG. *Problem Solving in Musculoskeletal Imaging.* Philadelphia, PA: Mosby; 2008:336–339.

17 Answer B.   The majority of carpometacarpal (CMC) dislocations involve multiple joints. Dislocation of the CMC joints other than the thumb is rare. When CMC dislocation occurs, there is usually an associated fracture due to the strength of the CMC and intermetacarpal ligaments. The index (second) and long (third) finger CMC articulations are relatively immobile, and therefore ring (fourth) and little (fifth) finger CMC dislocations are more common. CMC dislocations can be subtle on the standard three radiographic views of the hand, and CT can be helpful when CMC dislocation is suspected.

Reference: Pope T, Harris J. *Harris and Harris' the Radiology of Emergency Medicine.* 5th ed. Philadelphia, PA: Lippincott Williams & Wilkins; 2013:433–436.

18 Answer A.   The shoulder is the most commonly dislocated joint in the body. Anterior dislocations are far more common than posterior. In the anterior infracoracoid dislocation subtype, the humeral head rests below the coracoid. This pattern is the most common type of dislocation. Dislocation frequently happens at the glenohumeral joint due to the large humeral head articular surface compared to that of the glenoid and due to the relative weakness of the capsule.

Reference: Pope TL, Harris JH. *Harris and Harris' the Radiology of Emergency Medicine.* 5th ed. Philadelphia, PA: Lippincott Williams & Wilkins; 2013:319–332.

19 Answer D.   The images demonstrate extensive edema at the anterior inferior iliac spine. The sagittal image shows no normal rectus femoris tendon fibers extending from the anterior inferior iliac spine. The rectus femoris muscle is a long fusiform muscle with two heads. The direct head originates from the anterior inferior iliac spine, and the indirect head originates from the superior acetabular ridge. Most rectus femoris injuries occur at the myotendinous junction. However, tears at the origin can occur in kicking injuries.

Reference: Gyftopoulos S, Rosenberg ZS, Schweitzer ME, et al. Normal anatomy and strains of the deep musculotendinous junction of the proximal rectus femoris: MRI features. *AJR Am J Roentgenol.* 2008;190:W182–W186.

20   Answer B.   The axial MR image of the knee demonstrates medial patellar facet and lateral femoral condyle bone contusions, as well as disruption of the medial patellofemoral retinaculum. These findings are consistent with the sequela of lateral patellar dislocation. Several risk factors for patellar instability have been identified, including trochlear dysplasia, patella alta, and lateralization of the tibial tuberosity. The medial retinaculum and medial patellofemoral ligament are the most important ligamentous stabilizers of the patella.

References: Diederichs G, Issever AS, Scheffler S. MR imaging of patellar instability: injury patterns and assessment of risk factors. *Radiographics.* 2010;30:961–981.
Elias DA, White LM, Fithian DC. Acute lateral patellar dislocation at MR imaging: injury patterns of medial patellar soft-tissue restraints and osteochondral injuries of the inferomedial patella. *Radiology.* 2002;225:736–743.

21   Answer D.   The lateral upright radiograph of the cervical spine shows an avulsion fracture of the C7 spinous process, called a clay shoveler's fracture. This injury occurs as a result of abrupt flexion of the head. The tensed interspinous ligaments of the posterior neck result in avulsion of the spinous process. The clay shoveler's fracture can occur at C6, C7, and T1. This fracture is mechanically and neurologically stable. Of note, the Anderson-D'Alonzo classification system describes fractures of the dens.

Reference: Pope TL, Harris JH. *Harris and Harris' the Radiology of Emergency Medicine.* 5th ed. Philadelphia, PA: Lippincott Williams & Wilkins; 2013:190.

22   Answer D.   Tears of the proximal myotendinous junction of the plantaris may result in a curvilinear fluid collection or hematoma located between the medial head of gastrocnemius and soleus muscles, as seen in the provided images. The lack of abnormal signal within the gastrocnemius and soleus muscles argues against injury to these structures. A dissecting popliteal cyst can be traced back to its origin between the tendons of the medial head of gastrocnemius muscle and the semimembranosus muscle at the level of the knee. Patients suffering from plantaris tendon injury may sense a "pop" followed by sudden-onset calf pain. Conservative management is the treatment of choice.

Reference: Stoller DW. *Magnetic Resonance Imaging in Orthopaedics and Sports Medicine.* 3rd ed. Philadelphia, PA: Lippincott Williams & Wilkins; 2007:006–009.

23   Answer B.   Luxatio erecta, or inferior dislocation of the glenohumeral joint, is a rare entity that accounts for ~0.5% of all shoulder dislocations. Although rare, it has a characteristic imaging and clinical presentation, with the shaft of the humerus externally rotated and directed cephalad. Luxatio erecta has a classic clinical presentation with the patient unable to move the arm at the shoulder. The arm is held above the head with the elbow flexed. This hyperabduction injury may result in rotator cuff tear, injury to the brachial plexus, and injury to the axillary artery or vein. Fractures of the greater tuberosity, acromion process, and inferior glenoid rim may also be associated with this injury.

References: Downey EF Jr, Curtis DJ, Brower AC. Unusual dislocations of the shoulder. *AJR Am J Roentgenol.* 1983;140:1207–1210.
Kothari K, Bernstein RM, Griffiths HJ, et al. Luxatio erecta. *Skeletal Radiol.* 1984;11:47–49.

24a Answer C.   The sagittal T2-weighted fat-saturated MR image demonstrates a full-thickness tear of the Achilles tendon. This injury commonly occurs in middle-aged "weekend warriors" participating in activities requiring sudden forceful plantar flexion. Several factors may predispose to this injury. Systemic disorders such as rheumatoid arthritis, diabetes, and crystalline arthropathies have a proven association with Achilles tendon tears. Of the medications linked to Achilles tendon rupture, steroids and fluoroquinolone antibiotics have the greatest association.

References: Morrison WB, Sanders TG. *Problem Solving in Musculoskeletal Imaging.* Philadelphia, PA: Mosby; 2008:662–666.
Sode J, Obel N, Hallas J, et al. Use of fluoroquinolone and risk of Achilles tendon rupture: a population-based cohort study. *Eur J Clin Pharmacol.* 2007;63:499–503.

24b Answer C.   In this case, disruption of the tendon has occurred in the most common location, the relatively avascular zone found 2 to 6 cm proximal to the calcaneal insertion.

References: Morrison WB, Sanders TG. *Problem Solving in Musculoskeletal Imaging.* Philadelphia, PA: Mosby; 2008:662–666.
Sode J, Obel N, Hallas J, et al. Use of fluoroquinolone and risk of Achilles tendon rupture: a population-based cohort study. *Eur J Clin Pharmacol.* 2007;63:499–503.

25 Answer A.   A Bennett fracture is a noncomminuted intra-articular fracture of the base of the thumb metacarpal. The larger fracture fragment is retracted proximally by the unopposed action of the abductor pollicis longus tendon. This injury may require open reduction and internal fixation. A Rolando fracture is a three-part intra-articular fracture of the first metacarpal base and has a worse prognosis than the two-part Bennett fracture.

References: Morrison WB, Sanders TG. *Problem Solving in Musculoskeletal Imaging.* Philadelphia, PA: Mosby; 2008:495–496.
Pope TL, Harris JH. *Harris and Harris' the Radiology of Emergency Medicine.* 5th ed. Philadelphia, PA: Lippincott Williams & Wilkins; 2013:429–431.

26 Answer A.   Acetabular labral detachments are more common than tears. Most acetabular labral tears are located anterosuperiorly. The anterior superior portion of the acetabular labrum may be affected by femoroacetabular impingement. Posterior acetabular labral tears are much less common and are usually seen in young and athletic patients.

Reference: Blankenbaker DG, Tuite MJ. Acetabular labrum. *Magn Reson Imaging Clin N Am.* 2013;21:21–33.

27 Answer D.   Several systems exist for classification of acetabular fracture, but the Judet-LeTournel system is the most widely accepted. This classification system uses the column principle of the acetabulum. The anterior column is longer and larger and extends from the superior pubic ramus to the iliac wing. The posterior column extends from the ischiopubic ramus to the ilium. There are 10 types of fractures in the Judet-LeTournel system, but the most common (90%) are the both column, T shaped, transverse, transverse with posterior wall, and isolated posterior wall. Both column and T shaped fractures disrupt the obturator ring, and only the both column fracture involves the iliac wing.

Reference: Durkee NJ, Jacobson J, Jamadar D, et al. Classification of common acetabular fractures: radiographic and CT appearances. *AJR Am J Roentgenol.* 2006;187:915–925.

28 Answer C.   When a patient is placed in abduction and external rotation (ABER), the anterior inferior glenohumeral ligament is under tension. This stress on the capsule and anteroinferior labroligamentous complex can produce separation of a tear that will fill with contrast, and thus will be better visualized than on routine neutral positioning.

Reference: Saleem AM, Lee JK, Novak LM. Usefulness of the abduction and external rotation views in shoulder MR arthrography. *AJR Am J Roentgenol.* 2008;191:1024–1030.

29 Answer A. The coronal proton density fat-saturated MR image demonstrates displaced meniscal tissue in the medial aspect of the intercondylar notch. The sagittal proton density MR image on the right demonstrates the double PCL sign with displaced meniscal tissue in the intercondylar notch. This patient has a bucket handle tear of the medial meniscus. Longitudinal tears, either vertical or horizontal, are the most common types of meniscal tears. In a bucket handle tear, the inner fragment of the torn meniscus is displaced toward the notch. The handle of the bucket is formed by the displaced meniscal fragment with the bucket formed by the peripheral nondisplaced meniscal component.

Reference: Resnick D, Kang HS, Pretterkieber ML. *Internal Derangement of Joints.* 2nd ed. Philadelphia, PA: Saunders; 2007:1657–1660.

30 Answer B. Injury to the acromioclavicular joint can be classified in regard to which stabilizing ligamentous structures are damaged. In grade I injuries, there is a sprain of the acromioclavicular ligament that is not evident radiographically. With a grade II injury, there is complete disruption of the acromioclavicular ligament resulting in widening of the joint space, typically regarded as exceeding 4 mm. Variable injury to the coracoclavicular ligament can be present in a grade II injury; however, complete disruption is not present. Both grade I and grade II injuries usually respond well to nonsurgical management and should be differentiated from a grade III injury, in which there is complete disruption of the coracoclavicular ligament. This thick and relatively strong ligamentous complex consists of two components: the trapezoid and the conoid. This injury is often evident clinically; however, this can be seen radiographically as elevation of the clavicle and an increased coracoclavicular distance. Some classification systems include additional grades IV–VI, which are beyond the scope of this discussion.

References: Morrison WB, Sanders TG. *Problem Solving in Musculoskeletal Imaging.* Philadelphia, PA: Mosby; 2008:338–339.
Pope TL, Harris JH. *Harris and Harris' the Radiology of Emergency Medicine.* 5th ed. Philadelphia, PA: Lippincott Williams & Wilkins; 2013:313–319.

31 Answer B. The frontal radiograph of the knee demonstrates a proximally retracted avulsion fracture of the fibular head, referred to as the arcuate sign. This injury has a high association with injury to the posterolateral corner of the knee. The posterolateral corner structures include the lateral collateral ligament, the fabellofibular ligament, the popliteofibular ligament, the arcuate ligament, the popliteal tendon, and the biceps femoris tendon. If left unrecognized, an injury to the posterolateral corner structures can result in chronic instability. This instability ultimately may lead to failure of anterior cruciate ligament reconstruction.

References: Huang GS, Yu JS, Munshi M et al. Avulsion fracture of the head of the fibula (the "arcuate" sign): MR imaging findings predictive of injuries to the posterolateral ligaments and posterior cruciate ligament. *AJR Am J Roentgenol.* 2003;180:381–387.
Strub WM. The arcuate sign. *Radiology.* 2007;244:620–621.

32 Answer B. The axillary view demonstrates posterior dislocation of the humeral head. Additional radiographic findings associated with posterior shoulder dislocation include impaction fracture of the anterior humeral head, opposite of the Hill-Sachs lesion associated with anterior shoulder dislocation in which impaction occurs posterolaterally. With posterior dislocation, the shoulder may be locked in extreme internal rotation on AP images. There may be increased distance between the articular cortex of the humeral head and glenoid known as the positive rim sign; however, the opposite can also occur in which this distance is decreased. A fracture of the posterior glenoid may also be seen, referred to as a reverse Bankart lesion.

Reference: Pope TL, Harris JH. *Harris and Harris' the Radiology of Emergency Medicine.* 5th ed. Philadelphia, PA: Lippincott Williams & Wilkins; 2013:326–332.

33   **Answer A.**   Gamekeeper thumb refers to an injury of the ulnar collateral ligament (UCL) at the thumb metacarpophalangeal joint (MCP). Currently, the injury is most frequently seen in skiing-related trauma. Mechanistically, the injury results from excessive valgus stress applied across the MCP joint of the thumb. The injury may be associated with avulsion fractures of the distal attachment of the ulnar collateral ligament, as pictured. MRI is often performed with suspected UCL injuries, both to evaluate the degree of injury to the UCL and to determine the presence or absence of a Stener lesion, which requires surgical management. A Stener lesion refers to cases in which the torn and retracted proximal UCL becomes entrapped superficial to the adductor aponeurosis, preventing apposition of the proximal and distal fragments and thus resulting in inadequate healing.

References: Morrison WB, Sanders TG. *Problem Solving in Musculoskeletal Imaging.* Philadelphia, PA: Mosby; 2008:491.
Pope TL, Harris JH. *Harris and Harris' the Radiology of Emergency Medicine.* 5th ed. Philadelphia, PA: Lippincott Williams & Wilkins; 2013:431–423.

34   **Answer C.**   Sagittal proton density and proton density fat-saturated images of the knee demonstrate an abnormal band of hypointense tissue within the posterior intercondylar notch anterior to and paralleling the posterior cruciate ligament, the so-called double PCL sign. This finding is seen in the setting of a bucket handle tear of the medial meniscus with meniscal tissue displaced into the posterior intercondylar notch. When a bucket handle tear occurs laterally, which is less common, the double PCL sign does not typically occur because the ACL blocks the fragment from entering the posterior notch. This case also demonstrates a classic example of the double delta or double anterior horn, which represents a bucket handle tear with meniscal tissue flipped anteriorly into the intercondylar notch.

Reference: Morrison WB, Sanders TG. *Problem Solving in Musculoskeletal Imaging.* Philadelphia, PA: Mosby; 2008:601–604.

35   **Answer E.**   Stress injuries/fractures of bone can be classified on MRI by a five-point system as follows:

Grade 0: Normal study
Grade 1: Subtle periosteal edema
Grade 2: Periosteal edema in addition to marrow edema on T2-weighted fat-saturated images
Grade 3: More extensive periosteal edema; marrow changes on both T2-weighted fat-saturated and T1-weighted sequences
Grade 4: True stress fractures with a fracture line visible on MRI or radiographs

Reference: Hwang B, Fredericson M, Chung CB, et al. MRI findings of femoral diaphyseal stress injuries in athletes. *AJR Am J Roentgenol.* 2005;185:166–173.

36   **Answer C.**   Knee dislocations are defined based upon the location of the tibia with respect to the femur. Knee dislocation is a true orthopedic emergency due to the high association with vascular injury. The popliteal artery, being relatively fixed, is prone to stretch injury or laceration, with resultant thrombosis. This limb-threatening injury, if not managed based on clinical findings, requires rapid diagnosis. CT angiography is readily available in most emergency departments, is fast, and offers the added benefit of identifying additional osseous injuries that may not be evident radiographically. While MRI with contrast could potentially identify a vascular injury, the long time required to obtain the needed sequences prohibits its use in such situations. In the setting of knee dislocation when vascular injury has been excluded, MRI almost invariably shows disruption of both anterior and posterior cruciate ligaments in addition to various capsular injuries.

Reference: Pope TL, Harris JH. *Harris and Harris' the Radiology of Emergency Medicine.* 5th ed. Philadelphia, PA: Lippincott Williams & Wilkins; 2013:876.

37a Answer D. A frontal radiograph of the left ankle demonstrates a 4-mm talar dome osteochondral lesion. This lesion often occurs as the result of inversion injury and may involve the medial or lateral talar dome. MRI is the modality of choice for characterizing these lesions, including estimating stability.

References: Morrison WB, Sanders TG. *Problem Solving in Musculoskeletal Imaging.* Philadelphia, PA: Mosby; 2008:685–687.
Pope TL, Harris JH. *Harris and Harris' the Radiology of Emergency Medicine.* 5th ed. Philadelphia, PA: Lippincott Williams & Wilkins; 2013:953.

37b Answer A. Findings indicating instability include fluid signal surrounding the fragment, cystic change underneath the fragment, and frank displacement. The addition of intra-articular contrast may help to differentiate granulation tissue surrounding a healing injury from actual fluid, which would indicate instability.

References: Morrison WB, Sanders TG. *Problem Solving in Musculoskeletal Imaging.* Philadelphia, PA: Mosby; 2008:685–687.
Pope TL, Harris JH. *Harris and Harris' the Radiology of Emergency Medicine.* 5th ed. Philadelphia, PA: Lippincott Williams & Wilkins; 2013:953.

38 Answer A. The volar plate is a thickened, fibrous band of connective tissue along the palmar aspect of the first metacarpophalangeal and second through fifth interphalangeal joint capsules. This structure combines with the radial and ulnar collateral ligaments to maintain stability across these joints. The volar plate is most commonly injured at the level of the PIP joint and results from hyperextension. In some cases, the volar plate avulses a thin fragment of bone from the palmar aspect of the base of the middle phalanx, as pictured in the lateral radiograph. This injury is best appreciated on lateral images of the digit of concern.

References: Morrison WB, Sanders TG. *Problem Solving in Musculoskeletal Imaging.* Philadelphia, PA: Mosby; 2008:477–478.
Pope TL, Harris JH. *Harris and Harris' the Radiology of Emergency Medicine.* 5th ed. Philadelphia, PA: Lippincott Williams & Wilkins; 2013:427–428.

39 Answer B. The provided images demonstrate an elbow joint effusion with a fat pad or sail sign on the lateral view. No fracture is evident. The anterior and posterior fat pads of the elbow are intracapsular and extrasynovial. In a normal elbow, the anterior fat pad is a subtle linear lucency that parallels the anterior distal humerus. The normal posterior fat pad is usually not visualized as it is pressed into the olecranon fossa. When the elbow joint is distended, there is displacement of the fat pads as long as the joint capsule is intact. In the setting of trauma, a displaced anterior and/or posterior fat pad with no fracture should raise the clinical suspicion of an occult fracture. Distention of the fat pads is independent of fracture comminution or displacement. In the emergent setting,

CT is the most appropriate imaging study to evaluate for an occult fracture. Stress views may be painful for the patient and are unlikely to detect subtle fractures. MRI is costly and time consuming and may not be readily available in the emergent setting. Subtle fractures can be difficult to identify on ultrasound in the hands of radiologists unfamiliar with musculoskeletal ultrasound.

Reference: Goswami GK. The fat pad sign. *Radiology.* 2002;222:419–420.

40 Answer B.   An axial proton density fat-saturated image of the upper leg demonstrates edema within the anterior compartment musculature, specifically within the tibialis anterior and extensor digitorum longus muscles. In this particular case, these findings represented denervation secondary to traumatic injury to the peroneal nerve. This injury most commonly occurs at the level of the fibular head, where the nerve is prone to direct trauma. If no history of trauma is present, one must search for causes of extrinsic nerve compression including ganglia and other masses centered about the proximal tibiofibular joint. The peroneal nerve arises from the sciatic nerve in the thigh and travels posterior to the biceps femoris, ultimately coursing lateral to the fibular head. It provides innervation to the peroneus longus and brevis, tibialis anterior, extensor hallucis longus, extensor digitorum longus, and peroneus tertius. Injury can result in loss of strength in ankle dorsiflexors, the so-called foot drop.

Reference: Sonin A, Manaster BJ, Andrews CL, et al. *Diagnostic Imaging: Musculoskeletal: Trauma.* Manitoba, Canada: Amirsys; 2010:6:207.

41 Answer C.   Fracture healing is a complex process. Within 10 to 14 days of the fracture, the fracture line widens and the margins of the fracture fragments begin to blur. Then callus appears about the fracture site. The callus eventually fills in with bridging of the fracture line by calcified callus.

Reference: Rogers LF. *Radiology of Skeletal Trauma.* 3rd ed. New York, NY: Churchill Livingstone; 2001:209.

42 Answer C.   An oblique radiograph of the foot shows a small avulsion fracture arising from the fifth metatarsal base. This injury results from inversion of the plantar flexed foot. The classic teaching is that this fracture results from avulsion of the peroneus brevis attachment at the fifth metatarsal base; however, avulsion of the lateral component of the plantar aponeurosis can also produce this appearance.

References: Pope TL, Harris JH. *Harris and Harris' the Radiology of Emergency Medicine.* 5th ed. Philadelphia, PA: Lippincott Williams & Wilkins; 2013:958–959.
Theodorou DJ, Theodorou SJ, Kakitsubata Y, et al. Fractures of proximal portion of fifth metatarsal bone: anatomic and imaging evidence of a pathogenesis of avulsion of the plantar aponeurosis and the short peroneal muscle tendon. *Radiology.* 2003;226:857–865.

43a Answer A.   The coronal T2-weighted fat-saturated image shows a full-thickness rotator cuff tear with proximal tendinous retraction to the level of the medial humeral head and superior humeral migration. The oblique sagittal images demonstrate atrophy and fatty infiltration of the infraspinatus, as well as supraspinatus muscle volume loss. The teres minor and subscapularis muscles appear relatively normal in signal and volume on these images.

Reference: Sonin A, Manaster BJ, Andrews CL, et al. *Diagnostic Imaging: Musculoskeletal: Trauma.* Manitoba, Canada: Amirsys; 2010:2:78–83.

43b Answer A.   Listed in order from greatest to least frequency, rotator cuff tears most commonly involve the supraspinatus, followed by infraspinatus, subscapularis, and teres minor.

Reference: Sonin A, Manaster BJ, Andrews CL, et al. *Diagnostic Imaging: Musculoskeletal: Trauma.* Manitoba, Canada: Amirsys; 2010:2:78–83.

44 **Answer B.** The 3D CT images show a spiral fracture of the distal fibula, a fracture of the posterior malleolus, and a transverse fracture of the medial malleolus. These imaging findings are compatible with a supination external rotation injury, which is the most common Lauge-Hansen mechanism and is estimated to account for 40% to 70% of all ankle fractures. The spiral fibular fracture helps to identify this injury and demonstrates a low anterior to high posterior orientation. Once the fibular fracture is evident, the injury is considered to be stage II. Associated fractures of the posterior and medial malleoli (or injury to the deltoid ligamentous complex) further categorize these fractures as stage III and stage IV injuries, respectively. In the provided case, the medial malleolar fracture makes this a supination–external rotation stage IV injury.

Reference: Okanobo H, Khurana B, Sheehan S, et al. Simplified diagnostic algorithm for Lauge-Hansen classification of ankle injuries. *Radiographics.* 2012;32:E71–E84.

45 **Answer B.** The axial CT image demonstrates the classic reverse hamburger bun sign, in which the normally nonarticulating convex surfaces of the facets articulate with one another. This unstable injury results from hyperflexion, causing anterior and superior displacement of the inferior articulating process over the superior articulating process of the subjacent vertebra. This finding is best appreciated on sagittal reformats. Bilateral interfacetal dislocation is associated with extensive ligamentous injury and anterolisthesis of the more superior vertebral body, producing compromise of the spinal canal. MRI should be performed to evaluate the extent of ligamentous and spinal cord injury. Some discourage the use of the phrase "bilateral locked facets" in this injury, as the word "locked" implies a stable injury.

Reference: Pope TL, Harris JH. *Harris and Harris' the Radiology of Emergency Medicine.* 5th ed. Philadelphia, PA: Lippincott Williams & Wilkins; 2013:171, 184–188.

46 **Answer D.** On MRI, medial collateral ligament injuries can be classified as grades I–III. In grade I, the ligament is sprained with fluid superficial to the ligament. The ligament is partially torn in grade II injuries and completely torn with grade III injuries. Chronic injury to the MCL results in a thickened ligament. Pellegrini-Stieda refers to ossification of the medial collateral ligament in the setting of chronic injury.

Reference: Morrison WB, Sanders TG. *Problem Solving in Musculoskeletal Imaging.* Philadelphia, PA: Mosby; 2008:589–593.

47a **Answer B.** The pelvic radiograph demonstrates a subtle fracture of the left posterior wall of the acetabulum.

Reference: Pope TL, Harris JH. *Harris and Harris' the Radiology of Emergency Medicine.* 5th ed. Philadelphia, PA: Lippincott Williams & Wilkins; 2013:834–836.

47b **Answer B.** On MRI, there is a moderate left hip effusion and a mildly displaced fracture of the left posterior acetabular wall. These findings are consistent with prior posterior hip dislocation. When the femoral head dislocates posteriorly, the posterior rim of the acetabulum may be fractured. Posterior hip dislocations are more common than anterior dislocations. Femoral head fractures are common in the setting of hip dislocations.

Reference: Pope TL, Harris JH. *Harris and Harris' the Radiology of Emergency Medicine.* 5th ed. Philadelphia, PA: Lippincott Williams & Wilkins; 2013:834–836.

48 **Answer D.** The soft tissue defects along the lateral aspects of the fifth metatarsal heads bilaterally represent electrical exit wounds. The patient ultimately required amputation at the level of the fifth ray metatarsals bilaterally. Thermal trauma may have various radiologic manifestations including acroosteolysis, soft tissue wounds, myonecrosis, and dystrophic calcifications. Frostbite often spares the thumb, as the clenched fist position protects the thumb distal phalanx. The small vessels supplying the physes in skeletally immature patients are vulnerable to thermal trauma, which may manifest as premature physeal closure and limb length discrepancies. Fatty atrophy of musculature may result from thermal trauma, which is manifested by volume loss and increased T1-weighted MR signal (T1 shortening).

Reference: Crouch C, Smith WL. Long term sequelae of frostbite. *Pediatr Radiol.* 1990;20:365–366.

49 Answer A.   Essex-Lopresti is the name given to an injury consisting of a radial head fracture in conjunction with disruption of the distal radioulnar joint (DRUJ). The ulna is usually dorsally subluxed or dislocated at the DRUJ in this injury. The radial head fracture is usually comminuted. A Monteggia fracture consists of an ulnar diaphyseal fracture combined with dislocation of the radial head at the radiocapitellar joint. Galeazzi is the named injury that combines a distal radial shaft fracture with disruption of the DRUJ. A nightstick fracture refers to an isolated, typically nondisplaced fracture of the ulnar diaphysis.

Reference: Pope TL, Harris JH. *Harris and Harris' the Radiology of Emergency Medicine.* 5th ed. Philadelphia, PA: Lippincott Williams & Wilkins; 2013:366.

50 Answer A.   The scaphoid has a variable blood supply. However, 70% to 80% of patients have a distal blood supply with a branch that supplies the proximal pole. Scaphoid waist fractures can disrupt the blood supply to the middle and proximal poles. The more proximal the fracture in the scaphoid, the higher the incidence of avascular necrosis due to disruption of blood supply.

Reference: Pope TL, Harris JH. *Harris and Harris' the Radiology of Emergency Medicine.* 5th ed. Philadelphia, PA: Lippincott Williams & Wilkins; 2013:398–403.

51a Answer C.   The frontal knee radiograph demonstrates a small avulsion fracture arising from the lateral rim of the tibia at the lateral capsular attachment site, posterior to Gerdy tubercle. The Segond fracture has a >90% association with anterior cruciate ligament pathology and results from forced internal rotation of the flexed knee.

Reference: Pope TL, Harris JH. *Harris and Harris' the Radiology of Emergency Medicine.* 5th ed. Philadelphia, PA: Lippincott Williams & Wilkins; 2013:881–884.

51b Answer D.   A mirror image injury, avulsion of the medial tibial rim at the attachment of the deep capsular component of the medial collateral ligament, can also occur. This injury, known as the reverse Segond fracture, has a high association with injury to the posterior cruciate ligament and medial meniscus.

Reference: Pope TL, Harris JH. *Harris and Harris' the Radiology of Emergency Medicine.* 5th ed. Philadelphia, PA: Lippincott Williams & Wilkins; 2013:881–884.

52 Answer D.   Proximal femur fractures can be classified as intracapsular or extracapsular. Intracapsular fractures include subcapital, transcervical, and basicervical. Examples of extracapsular fractures include intertrochanteric, subtrochanteric, and trochanteric. Intracapsular fractures are much more susceptible to femoral head avascular necrosis with an incidence of 10% to 35%. If the fracture is subcapital and is significantly displaced, there is a 66% to 88% incidence of avascular necrosis of the fragment as a result of disruption of blood flow to the femoral head fragment.

Reference: Pope TL, Harris JH. *Harris and Harris' the Radiology of Emergency Medicine.* 5th ed. Philadelphia, PA: Lippincott Williams & Wilkins; 2013:836–843.

53 Answer D. The axially view of the shoulder demonstrates an unfused acromion process, or os acromiale. The acromion should fuse between the ages of 22 and 25 years. If the acromion remains unfused, it can result in rotator cuff impingement secondary to downward displacement during deltoid contraction. An os acromiale can mimic a fracture. The unfused acromion usually has a triangular appearance and has a sclerotic margin. The synchondrosis is always perpendicular to the long axis of the acromion. Acute fractures will usually have nonsclerotic margins and will be oblique with respect to the long axis of the acromion. There are four subtypes of os acromiale: basiacromion, meta-acromion, mesoacromion, and preacromion (from proximal to distal). Mesoacromion and meta-acromion are more common. If the os acromiale is mobile and unstable, there may be associated AC joint degenerative change.

References: Morrison WB, Sanders TG. *Problem Solving in Musculoskeletal Imaging.* Philadelphia, PA: Mosby; 2008:330–335.
Stoller DW. *Magnetic Resonance Imaging in Orthopaedics and Sports Medicine.* 3rd ed. Philadelphia, PA: Lippincott Williams & Wilkins; 2007:1241–1243.

54 Answer B. The image demonstrates abnormal edema in the left adductor musculature. The adductor longus tendon on the left is avulsed from its insertion on the pubic symphysis. The right adductor longus insertion is abnormally thickened. The patient had prior adductor longus repair on the right side. Athletic pubalgia is a difficult clinical diagnosis. There are multiple overlapping pathologies in the hip and groin region. In patients with clinical athletic pubalgia, the most common injuries are at the lateral border of the rectus abdominis slightly cephalad to its pubic attachment or at the origin of the rectus abdominis. A spectrum of injuries can be seen from partial tearing at the rectus abdominis–adductor longus aponeurosis to complete avulsion of the adductor longus tendon.

Reference: Omar IM, Zoga AC, Kavanagh EC, et al. Athletic pubalgia and "sports hernia": optimal MR imaging technique and findings. *Radiographics.* 2008;28:1415–1438.

55 Answer E. Posterior interosseous nerve syndrome is also known as deep radial nerve syndrome and supinator syndrome. Posterior interosseous nerve syndrome (PIN) presents with forearm pain, a nonspecific symptom. Some patients complain of weakness of the extensor muscles. Sensation is usually preserved. Posterior interosseous nerve syndrome is the result of radial nerve entrapment or compression at the supinator muscle. MRI typically shows denervation edema or atrophy of the involved muscles with sparing of the extensor carpi radialis longus. The most common site of nerve compression is the arcade of Frohse at the proximal edge of the supinator muscle. The most common MRI finding associated with posterior interosseous nerve syndrome is denervation edema or atrophy of the supinator or extensor muscles, which can indicate the level of the nerve lesion. The extensor carpi radialis longus muscle is classically spared.

References: Andreisek G, Crook DW, Burg D, et al. Peripheral neuropathies of the median, radial, and ulnar nerves: MR imaging features. *Radiographics.* 2006;26:1267–1287.
Miller TT, Reinus WR. Nerve entrapment syndromes of the elbow, forearm, and wrist. *AJR Am J Roentgenol.* 2010;195:585–594.

56 Answer B. A lateral radiograph of the knee shows thickening of the proximal patellar tendon, which contains tiny areas of internal dystrophic calcification. A sagittal proton density fat-saturated MR image demonstrates a thickened and inflamed patellar tendon with trace adjacent patellar and infrapatellar edema. Jumper's knee refers to proximal patellar tendinopathy, which results from repetitive overloading of the extensor mechanism, commonly experienced by jumping athletes such as basketball or volleyball players. Hoffa syndrome also results from repetitive microtrauma, but manifests as anterior knee pain with edema or fibrosis centered within the infrapatellar fat pad. Tennis leg is a term that describes an athletic injury characterized by sudden onset mid-calf pain associated with a "popping" sensation. While this injury had originally been attributed to rupture of the plantaris tendon, more recent studies have shown that injury to the medial head of gastrocnemius is more commonly associated with this clinical scenario.

References: Delgado GJ, Chung CB, Lektrakul N, et al. Tennis leg: clinical US study of 141 patients and anatomic investigation of four cadavers with MR imaging and US. *Radiology.* 2002;224:112–119.
Sonin A, Manaster BJ, Andrews CL, et al. *Diagnostic Imaging: Musculoskeletal: Trauma.* Manitoba, Canada: Amirsys; 2010:6:169; 7:137.

57 **Answer C.** The images show a linear echogenic foreign body in the lateral elbow soft tissues. The foreign body is surrounded by hypoechoic vascular material. There is clean posterior acoustic shadowing associated with the foreign body. The patient reported a remote history of scraping his elbow against a tree. The foreign body was a small splinter. Metallic, stone, and glass foreign bodies are usually apparent on radiographs. Wooden foreign bodies may not be visible on radiographs. Linear wooden foreign bodies commonly show posterior acoustic shadowing as depicted in the provided images. In the provided case, the splinter was surrounded by granulation tissue.

References: Horton LK, Jacobson JA, Powell A, et al. Sonography and radiography of soft-tissue foreign bodies. *AJR Am J Roentgenol.* 2001;176:1155–1159.
Peterson JJ, Bancroft LW, Kransdorf MJ. Wooden foreign bodies: imaging appearance. *AJR Am J Roentgenol.* 2002;178(3):557–562.

58 **Answer A.** A lateral radiograph of the hand demonstrates a proximally displaced avulsion fracture of the dorsal aspect of the base of the little finger distal phalanx. This represents the attachment site of the extensor tendon, which, in the case of the fifth finger, is named the extensor digiti minimi. Flexion deformity results from the unopposed action of the flexor digitorum profundus, which inserts volarly. This injury is known in the literature as both mallet finger and baseball finger. In some instances, the fracture occurs distal to the extensor insertion. In such cases, the fragment is not displaced proximally and no flexion deformity occurs.

References: Morrison WB, Sanders TG. *Problem Solving in Musculoskeletal Imaging.* Philadelphia, PA: Mosby; 2008:488–489.
Pope TL, Harris JH. *Harris and Harris' the Radiology of Emergency Medicine.* 5th ed. Philadelphia, PA: Lippincott Williams & Wilkins; 2013:425–427.

59a **Answer A.** Axial MR images of the shoulder and proximal humerus show evidence of complete proximal long head of biceps tendon rupture with an empty bicipital groove. The torn and distally retracted biceps tendon is surrounded by an edematous biceps muscle.

References: Morrison WB, Sanders TG. *Problem Solving in Musculoskeletal Imaging.* Philadelphia, PA: Mosby; 2008:412.
Sonin A, Manaster BJ, Andrews CL, et al. *Diagnostic Imaging: Musculoskeletal: Trauma.* Manitoba, Canada: Amirsys; 2010:2:106–109.

59b **Answer B.** The long head of biceps tendon originates from the biceps labral anchor at the supraglenoid tubercle and inserts distally on the radial tuberosity. Less than 5% of biceps tendon ruptures occur distally at the radial tuberosity. Proximal rupture is far more common and most often involves the intra-articular portion of the tendon. This injury most commonly occurs as an acute injury superimposed on a background of chronic tendinopathy in older patients. Patients may feel a "pop" followed by sudden relief of pain when a chronic partial tear is completed.

References: Morrison WB, Sanders TG. *Problem Solving in Musculoskeletal Imaging.* Philadelphia, PA: Mosby; 2008:412.
Sonin A, Manaster BJ, Andrews CL, et al. *Diagnostic Imaging: Musculoskeletal: Trauma.* Manitoba, Canada: Amirsys; 2010:2:106–109.

60 **Answer B.**   The axillary radiograph demonstrates a Hill-Sachs fracture, an impaction fracture of the posterolateral humeral head. The axial T2-weighted fat-saturated MR image is distal to the Hill-Sachs fracture, but the anteroinferior glenoid labrum is absent with medialized labral tissue along the anterior aspect of the glenoid. This imaging appearance is consistent with an anterior labroligamentous periosteal sleeve avulsion. The labral injury is a result of the humeral head contacting the labrum during dislocation. When the posterior humeral head impacts the glenoid labrum, the Hill-Sachs fracture occurs. Hill-Sachs fractures can occur without dislocation; any impaction on the posterior humerus can cause a fracture. However, there is a high association with dislocation and Hill-Sachs fracture, and for this reason, the anteroinferior labroligamentous complex should be scrutinized for injury on MRI when there is an impaction fracture or contusion of the posterolateral humeral head.

Reference: Pope TL, Harris JH. *Harris and Harris' the Radiology of Emergency Medicine.* 5th ed. Philadelphia, PA: Lippincott Williams & Wilkins; 2013:320–325.

61 **Answer B.**   A frontal radiograph of the right femur shows a displaced diaphyseal fracture. A coronal reformatted image from a contrast-enhanced abdomen/pelvis CT demonstrates a large filling defect within the inferior vena cava, portions of which have attenuation values of fat. Fat emboli most commonly occur following long bone fractures or intramedullary rod placement. CT imaging findings are usually nonspecific and may include peripheral ground-glass opacities, centrilobular nodules, and pulmonary edema. Actual macroscopic fat emboli, as seen in the provided case, are quite rare. VQ scan may demonstrate multiple, small, peripheral, subsegmental perfusion defects in the setting of fat embolism. Diagnosis is usually based upon clinical findings, which may include the triad of hypoxia, petechial rash, and altered mental status following a long bone fracture.

References: Arakawa H, Kurihara Y, Nakajima Y. Pulmonary fat embolism syndrome: CT findings in six patients. *J Comput Assist Tomogr.* 2000;24:24–29.
Parisi DM, Koval K, Egol K. Fat embolism syndrome. *Am J Orthop (Belle Mead NJ).* 2001;31:507–512.

62 **Answer C.**   A sagittal T2-weighted fat-saturated MR image demonstrates a fluid-filled gap in the expected location of the sesamoid–phalangeal ligament of the tibial hallux sesamoid, also known as injury of the plantar plate or turf toe. The sesamoid has migrated proximally in the provided example. This injury is the result of hyperextension at the metatarsophalangeal joint and occurs most frequently at this location in athletes involved in sports requiring rapid directional change. The name turf toe surfaced as a result of the fact that the injury was originally seen more frequently when harder, artificial playing surfaces were utilized. The intersesamoid ligament is not visualized on the provided image and would be best evaluated on axial sequences. The intact flexor hallucis longus tendon is seen on this image superficial to the disrupted sesamoid–phalangeal ligament.

References: Morrison WB, Sanders TG. *Problem Solving in Musculoskeletal Imaging.* Philadelphia, PA: Mosby; 2008:721–723.
Sonin A, Manaster BJ, Andrews CL, et al. *Diagnostic Imaging: Musculoskeletal: Trauma.* Manitoba, Canada: Amirsys; 2010:7:18–20.

63 **Answer B.** Coronal and axial proton density fat-saturated MR images demonstrate soft tissue edema between the iliotibial band and lateral femoral condyle, findings compatible with iliotibial band friction syndrome. This condition commonly manifests as anterolateral knee pain in long-distance runners and cyclists and results from repetitive contact between the IT band and lateral femoral condyle. The radiologist must carefully scrutinize the images to ensure that the signal abnormality does not simply represent normal joint fluid extending superiorly into the lateral knee joint recess. Additional findings may include lateral femoral condyle reactive bone marrow edema and abnormal signal within the IT band. Management is conservative, with most patients responding well to rest. The provided images show no evidence of IT band discontinuity, bone contusion, or vastus lateralis muscular tear.

Reference: Sonin A, Manaster BJ, Andrews CL, et al. *Diagnostic Imaging: Musculoskeletal: Trauma*. Manitoba, Canada: Amirsys; 2010:6:104–107.

64 **Answer D.** The glenoid labrum is typically divided into quadrants. Anatomic variants of the labrum occur in the anterosuperior labrum. A sublabral foramen is an anterosuperior labrum, which is unattached to the glenoid. If an MR arthrogram is performed or there is a large glenohumeral joint effusion, fluid can extend between the glenoid and labrum. A Buford complex refers to an absent or diminutive anterosuperior labrum with a thickened or cord-like middle glenohumeral ligament. A sublabral/superior recess is similar to a sublabral foramen except that the superior labrum is partially detached. Of the three variants described above, the sublabral/superior recess is most common occurring in ~75% of people. The sublabral foramen and Buford complex are much less common occurring in 10% and 1% to 2% of people, respectively. When interpreting a shoulder MRI, it is important to consider anatomic variants in the anterosuperior quadrant of the glenoid labrum.

Reference: Sonin A, Manaster BJ, Andrews CL, et al. *Diagnostic Imaging: Musculoskeletal: Trauma*. Manitoba, Canada: Amirsys; 2010:2:114–117.

65 **Answer B.** Carpal dislocations can be difficult to diagnose on radiographs. The most common form of carpal dislocation is perilunate dislocation. On the AP view, the lunate is triangular in shape. On the lateral view, there is volar rotation of the lunate with dorsal dislocation of the carpus with respect to the lunate. In lunate dislocation, as shown in the provided images, the lunate also has a triangular shape on the AP view, but the lunate is completely dislocated on the lateral view. The remainder of the carpus is normally aligned. The most common type of perilunate injury is transscaphoid perilunate dislocation where there is a scaphoid fracture and perilunate dislocation. The scaphocapitate fracture is a rare transverse fracture of the scaphoid waist and capitate that can occur with perilunate dislocation.

References: Kaewlai R, Avery LL, Ashwin AV, et al. Multidetector CT of carpal injuries: anatomy, fractures, and fracture-dislocations. *Radiographics*. 2008;28:1771–1784.
Pope TL, Harris JH. *Harris and Harris' the Radiology of Emergency Medicine*. 5th ed. Philadelphia, PA: Lippincott Williams & Wilkins; 2013:413–416.

66 **Answer B.** Fractures or bone loss involving the anterior inferior glenoid can result in chronic glenohumeral instability and repeated anterior shoulder dislocation. 3D CT has emerged as a useful means of quantifying glenoid bone deficiency, which can assist the surgeon in determining appropriate management. Generally, loss of >25% glenoid surface area indicates the need for surgical management. Alternatively, loss of >25% glenoid width based upon a best fit circle outlining the inferior glenoid can be used as a cutoff. The glenoid can be surgically restored via open reduction and internal fixation or bone grafting from various donor sites.

Reference: Bhatia S, Ghodadra NS, Romeo AA, et al. The importance of the recognition and treatment of glenoid bone loss in an athletic population. *Sports Health*. 2011;3:435–40.

67 **Answer D.**   Sagittal proton density and proton density fat-saturated MR images of the knee show full-thickness rupture of the distal quadriceps tendon. In the setting of acute full-thickness tears, early surgical repair is indicated. Quadriceps tears most frequently involve the tendon of the vastus intermedius. As a result of quadriceps tendon rupture, radiographs may show patella baja and avulsion fractures arising from the superior patella. Quadriceps rupture is relatively rare and most commonly occurs in patients with underlying conditions resulting in tendon weakening such as chronic renal disease, rheumatoid arthritis, or steroid use.

Reference: Sonin A, Manaster BJ, Andrews CL, et al. *Diagnostic Imaging: Musculoskeletal: Trauma*. Manitoba, Canada: Amirsys; 2010:6:162–164.

68a **Answer C.**   An enthesophyte describes bone proliferation at an enthesis, which denotes a site of tendon or ligament insertion onto bone. Enthesopathy is common and can result from chronic degeneration/overuse or with certain inflammatory arthropathies. An osteophyte refers to bone proliferation at a joint and is characteristic of degenerative arthrosis. The osteochondroses are a group of conditions affecting the apophyses and epiphyses of the immature skeleton and range from injuries resulting from repetitive microtrauma or avascular necrosis to normal asymptomatic variants.

References: Doyle SM, Monahan A. Osteochondroses: a clinical review for the pediatrician. *Curr Opin Pediatr.* 2010;22:41–46.
Sonin A, Manaster BJ, Andrews CL, et al. *Diagnostic Imaging: Musculoskeletal: Trauma*. Manitoba, Canada: Amirsys; 2010:7:172–173.

68b **Answer C.**   The images provided show Achilles tendon and plantar fascia insertional enthesophytes, with enlargement of the posterior process of the calcaneus and retrocalcaneal bursitis. This constellation of findings is referred to as the Haglund syndrome and presents with posterior calcaneal pain, often made worse by plantar flexion. Sever disease refers to an osteochondrosis involving the immature calcaneal apophysis. The plantar fascia is intact without adjacent increased T2 signal; therefore, plantar fasciitis is not seen. No stress fracture signal changes are noted in the calcaneus.

References: Doyle SM, Monahan A. Osteochondroses: a clinical review for the pediatrician. *Curr Opin Pediatr.* 2010;22:41–46.
Sonin A, Manaster BJ, Andrews CL, et al. *Diagnostic Imaging: Musculoskeletal: Trauma*. Manitoba, Canada: Amirsys; 2010:7:172–173.

69a **Answer C.**   Axial and sagittal T2-weighted fat-saturated MR images of the left thigh show fluid at the expected location of the tendinous origin of the hamstring muscles, at the ischial tuberosity. The gluteus medius arises from the ilium and inserts onto the lateral greater trochanter of the femur. The adductor longus arises from the anterior pubic bone and inserts on the medial lip of the linea aspera of the femur. The gluteus maximus arises in part from the posterior sacrum and coccyx and inserts onto the gluteal tuberosity of the femur. The iliopsoas arises in part from the iliac fossa and the sacral ala and inserts onto the lesser trochanter of the femur.

Reference: Koulouris G, Connell D. Hamstring muscle complex: an imaging review. *Radiographics.* 2005;25(3):571–586.

69b **Answer B.**   The hamstring muscles include the biceps femoris, semitendinosus, and semimembranosus. Each of these originates from the ischial tuberosity. The biceps femoris and semitendinosus begin as a conjoint tendon on the ischial tuberosity, posterior and medial relative to the semimembranosus. The semimembranosus, however, has a separate origin on the superior lateral facet of the ischial tuberosity, located more anterior and lateral on the tuberosity with respect to the biceps femoris and semitendinosus. The distally retracted semimembranosus tendon is well visualized on the sagittal image. The conjoint origin of the biceps femoris and semitendinosus is intact at the posterior ischial tuberosity, as seen on the axial image.

Reference: Koulouris G, Connell D. Hamstring muscle complex: an imaging review. *Radiographics.* 2005;25(3):571–586.

70 Answer D. The rotator interval is an area of the glenohumeral joint capsule that represents the space between the anterior margin of the supraspinatus tendon and the superior aspect of the subscapularis tendon. The coracohumeral ligament and superior glenohumeral ligament form the roof of the rotator interval and comprise the biceps tendon sling, which contains the intra-articular portion of the long head of biceps tendon. The structures of the rotator interval represent static stabilizers of the glenohumeral joint and biceps tendon; thus, injury to these structures can produce instability. Abnormal signal within the rotator interval is one of the several imaging findings, in addition to thickening of the axillary pouch, which can be associated with the clinical entity of adhesive capsulitis.

Reference: Morrison WB, Sanders TG. *Problem Solving in Musculoskeletal Imaging.* Philadelphia, PA: Mosby; 2008:360–364.

71 Answer A. The coronal T2-weighted fat-saturated MR images show fluid signal at the articular side of the common extensor origin indicating an intermediate-grade, partial-thickness tear consistent with lateral epicondylitis. The adjacent radial collateral ligament is intact on the coronal images. On the ulnar side of the joint, both the common flexor origin and the ulnar collateral ligament are intact. The common extensor tendon is composed of the extensor carpi radialis brevis, extensor digitorum communis, and extensor carpi ulnaris. The extensor carpi radialis brevis tendon is most commonly involved in lateral epicondylitis. On the medial side, the common flexor tendon is composed of the flexor carpi radialis, palmaris longus, and flexor carpi ulnaris. The flexor carpi ulnaris and pronator teres are most commonly involved in medial epicondylitis. MRI findings of epicondylitis include tendinosis with tendon thickening and increased signal intensity as well as tearing, which manifests as a fluid signal defect in the tendon. Tears can range from partial thickness to full thickness.

Reference: Walz DM, Newman JS, Konin GP, et al. Epicondylitis: pathogenesis, imaging, and treatment. *Radiographics.* 2010;30:167–184.

72 Answer D. Images demonstrate a large amount of fluid between the patella and overlying subcutaneous tissues. These findings are compatible with prepatellar bursitis or housemaid knee, which results from repetitive trauma to the anterior knee. The superficial infrapatellar bursa, known as preacher knee when inflamed, is located between the tibial tubercle and overlying skin. The deep infrapatellar bursa is located between the posterior patellar tendon and tibia. The suprapatellar bursa is located between the quadriceps tendon and the femur and communicates with the knee joint space. The pes anserine bursa separates the sartorius, gracilis, and semitendinosus tendons from the medial tibia and MCL.

References: Beaman FD, Peterson JJ. MR imaging of cysts, ganglia, and bursae about the knee. *Radiol Clin North Am.* 2007;45(6):969–982.

Lee P, Hunter TB, Taljanovic M. Musculoskeletal colloquialisms: how did we come up with these names? *Radiographics.* 2004;24:1009–1027.

73 Answer C. The axial T2-weighted MR image demonstrates a complete tear of the anterior inferior tibiofibular ligament. On the coronal T2-weighted MR image, fluid extends superiorly through a torn distal tibiofibular syndesmosis.

The syndesmotic ligamentous complex of the ankle is composed of the anterior inferior tibiofibular ligament, the posterior inferior tibiofibular ligament, inferior transverse tibiofibular ligament, and the inferior interosseous ligament/membrane. Due to its oblique course, the anterior inferior tibiofibular ligament is best visualized in the axial plane. Striations within the anterior inferior tibiofibular ligament are normal. Tears of the inferior tibiofibular ligaments can be partial or complete. Injury to the syndesmotic complex is also known as a high ankle injury.

Reference: Perrich KD, Goodwin DW, Hecht PJ, et al. Ankle ligaments on MRI: appearance of normal and injured ligaments. *AJR Am J Roentgenol.* 2009;193:687–95.

74 **Answer A.** The sagittal T2*-weighted gradient echo MR image of the knee shows a 13-mm femoral condyle osteochondritis dissecans. In this particular patient, the abnormality involves the lateral weight-bearing surface of the medial femoral condyle, the most common location in the adolescent knee. Osteochondritis dissecans is a term used in adolescents to describe a fracture extending through the articular cartilage and a portion of the underlying bone. Management of these lesions ranges from conservative to surgical and depends upon stability. It should be noted that the imaging criteria for instability differ among skeletally mature and skeletally immature individuals.

Reference: Sonin A, Manaster BJ, Andrews CL, et al. *Diagnostic Imaging: Musculoskeletal: Trauma.* Manitoba, Canada: Amirsys; 2010:6:46–51.

75 **Answer D.** The initial radiographs show a comminuted fracture of the radius that subsequently healed. The 6-week follow-up radiograph and CT scan demonstrate sclerosis of the proximal pole of the scaphoid consistent with avascular necrosis secondary to a scaphoid waist fracture. The osteopenia of the carpals is secondary to immobilization of wrist rather than reflex sympathetic dystrophy. There is no lucency around the fixation pins through the distal radius that would be expected in the case of hardware failure. Proximal pole scaphoid fractures are the most susceptible to avascular necrosis due to vascular disruption. Approximately 15% to 30% of scaphoid fractures develop avascular necrosis. The radiographic and CT findings include sclerosis, fragmentation, and collapse. The sclerotic bone demonstrates low T1 and fluid-sensitive signal intensity on MRI.

Reference: Sonin A, Manaster BJ, Andrews CL, et al. *Diagnostic Imaging: Musculoskeletal: Trauma.* Manitoba, Canada: Amirsys; 2010:4:44–49.

76a **Answer A.** The frontal radiograph shows loss of congruity of the carpal arcs and a triangular configuration of the lunate. The lateral view demonstrates maintenance of the expected alignment of the lunate and radius; however, the capitate and remaining carpal bones are dorsally dislocated. Findings are compatible with perilunate dislocation.

References: Pope TL, Harris JH. *Harris and Harris' the Radiology of Emergency Medicine.* 5th ed. Philadelphia, PA: Lippincott Williams & Wilkins; 2013:413–416.
Sonin A, Manaster BJ, Andrews CL, et al. *Diagnostic Imaging: Musculoskeletal: Trauma.* Manitoba, Canada: Amirsys; 2010:4:60–65.

76b **Answer C.** Lesser arc injuries are purely ligamentous injuries that progress through the carpal joint spaces in order of increasing severity as follows: (1) scapholunate (scapholunate dissociation), (2) lunocapitate (perilunate dislocation), (3) lunotriquetral (midcarpal dislocation), and (4) proximal migration of the capitate and unrestrained lunate (lunate dislocation).

References: Pope TL, Harris JH. *Harris and Harris' the Radiology of Emergency Medicine.* 5th ed. Philadelphia, PA: Lippincott Williams & Wilkins; 2013:413–416.
Sonin A, Manaster BJ, Andrews CL, et al. *Diagnostic Imaging: Musculoskeletal: Trauma.* Manitoba, Canada: Amirsys; 2010:4:60–65.

77 **Answer C.**   The images demonstrate extensive edema in the navicular with no fracture line visible. The most appropriate management in this patient with no fracture is conservative therapy as a first line of treatment. Immobilization and making the patient non–weight bearing will allow the bone marrow edema and stress reaction to resolve. Incomplete stress fractures (involving only one cortex) can also be managed with immobilization and non–weight bearing in some patients. In general, complete navicular stress fractures or sclerotic fractures will require surgical treatment with screw fixation of the fracture.

Reference: Berger FH, de Jonge MC, Maas M. Stress fractures in the lower extremity. The importance of increasing awareness amongst radiologists. *Eur J Radiol.* 2007;62:16–26.

78 **Answer B.**   The Gustilo open fracture classification system stratifies open fractures from grade I through grade IIIC based upon the size of the wound, the severity of associated soft tissue damage, and the presence or absence of wound contamination and arterial compromise. In the case provided, the mechanism indicates a contaminated wound, and probing of the wound showed extensive soft tissue injury. Many open tibial shaft fractures undergo intramedullary nail fixation; however, for those accompanied by extensive soft tissue damage or wound contamination, initial external fixation is the treatment of choice. External fixation can help to restore length and alignment, while protecting soft tissues from continued fracture fragment mobility. External fixation devices also facilitate access to the wound for inspection and debridement, which is crucial in cases of heavily contaminated injuries.

References: Cross WW, Swiontkowski MF. Treatment principles in the management of open fractures. *Indian J Orthop.* 2008;42:377–86.

Gustilo RB, Mendoza RM, Williams DN. Problems in the management of type III (severe) open fractures: a new classification of type III open fractures. *J Trauma.* 1984;24:742–746.

79 **Answer D.**   The images demonstrate a focal mass-like structure anterior to the anterior cruciate ligament graft. The mass is relatively low in signal intensity. This abnormality is the appearance of focal arthrofibrosis with a cyclops lesion. One of the presenting symptoms of arthrofibrosis is incomplete and/or painful knee extension because the nodule can become trapped between the femur and tibia. Arthrofibrosis can also be diffuse; however, the focal form is more common after anterior cruciate ligament reconstruction.

References: Meyers AB, Haims AH, Menn K, et al. Imaging of anterior cruciate ligament repair and its complications. *AJR Am J Roentgenol.* 2010;194:476–84.

Recht MP, Kramer J. MR imaging of the postoperative knee: a pictorial essay. *Radiographics.* 2002;22:765–74.

80 **Answer D.**   The MR images show contrast extending between the deep fibers of the distal ulnar collateral ligament and sublime tubercle of the ulna, a finding known as the T sign. This finding is diagnostic of a partial-thickness, articular side tear of the distal ulnar collateral ligament. This injury is seen as a result of repetitive or excessive valgus force upon the elbow, which is most commonly seen in high-performance throwing athletes. With extreme valgus loading during the late cocking phase of throwing, the UCL is the primary lateral stabilizing structure.

References: Morrison WB, Sanders TG. *Problem Solving in Musculoskeletal Imaging.* Philadelphia, PA: Mosby; 2008:420–424.

Sonin A, Manaster BJ, Andrews CL, et al. *Diagnostic Imaging: Musculoskeletal: Trauma.* Manitoba, Canada: Amirsys; 2010:3:62–67.

7

Metabolic and Hematologic Disorders

QUESTIONS

1   Looser zones in osteomalacia are typically located where in the femur?

   A. Femoral head
   B. Greater trochanter
   C. Lateral subtrochanteric region
   D. Medial subtrochanteric region

2a   Based on the images below, what is the most likely diagnosis in this 26-year-old female?

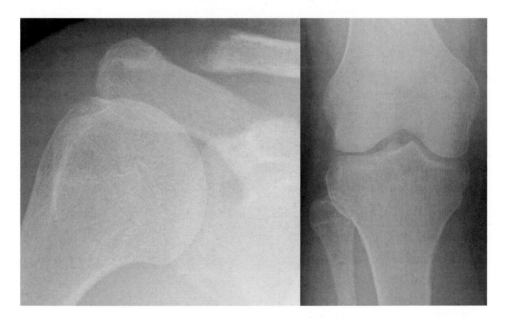

   A. Hyperthyroidism
   B. Hyperparathyroidism
   C. Hypothyroidism
   D. Hypoparathyroidism

2b What is the earliest radiographic finding of hyperparathyroidism?

A. Subperiosteal resorption of the medial cortex of the tibia
B. Subchondral resorption of the distal clavicle
C. Subligamentous resorption of the coracoclavicular ligament at the clavicular attachment
D. Subperiosteal resorption of the radial surface of the second and third digit middle phalanx

2c What percentage of cases of primary hyperparathyroidism results from a parathyroid adenoma?

A. 75% to 85%
B. 55% to 65%
C. 35% to 45%
D. 15% to 25%

3 In acromegaly, a heel pad thickness greater than how many centimeters is characteristic for a male?

A. 1.8 cm
B. 2.3 cm
C. 2.8 cm
D. 3.3 cm

4a A 75-year-old female with osteoporosis presents with pain in the right hip. What is most likely responsible for the finding below?

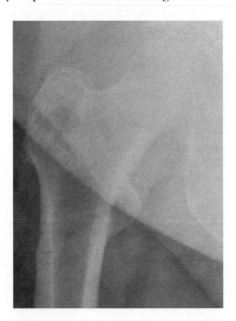

A. Looser zone
B. Bisphosphonate fracture
C. Traumatic fracture
D. Stress fracture

4b What is the next most appropriate test?

A. Radiograph of the left hip/femur
B. Radiograph of the thoracic/lumbar spine
C. MRI of the right hip/femur
D. MRI of the pelvis/sacroiliac joints

4c   What is the best imaging test to diagnose osteoporosis?

    A. Radiographic skeletal survey
    B. MRI of the sacrum
    C. DEXA scan
    D. MRI of the lumbar spine

5   A 58-year-old male with renal osteodystrophy presents with the following radiograph. What crystal is responsible for the calcifications?

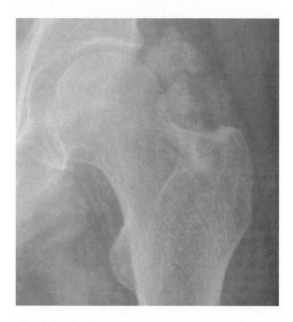

    A. Calcium pyrophosphate
    B. Uric acid
    C. Calcium hydroxyapatite
    D. Sodium urate

6   What is the most common location for periosteal new bone formation in thyroid acropachy?

    A. Tibia
    B. Humerus
    C. Distal phalanges
    D. Metacarpals

7   In myelofibrosis, which of the following is a characteristic bone marrow MRI appearance?

    A. T1-weighted bone marrow signal is lower than muscle or intervertebral disc signal.
    B. T2-weighted and STIR bone marrow signal is higher than normal.
    C. Bone marrow enhances on postcontrast images.
    D. Marrow signal drops out on opposed-phase imaging compared to in-phase imaging.

8   Which radiographic finding is seen in the setting of thalassemia?

    A. Thickened cortex that causes a "hair-on-end" appearance of the skull.
    B. Diffuse osteosclerosis of the bones of the axial skeleton.
    C. Widened medullary space of the tubular bones leads to absence of tubulation.
    D. Thinned horizontal trabeculae of the spine lead to a striated vertebral body appearance.

9a Based on the image below, what is the most likely cause of the visualized findings?

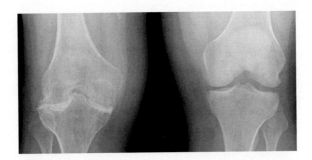

A. Chondrocalcinosis resulting from hyperparathyroidism
B. Chronic osteomyelitis associated with *S. aureus* infection
C. Disuse osteopenia resulting from a recent ipsilateral ankle fracture
D. Hemarthrosis in the joint resulting in synovitis

9b After the knee, what is the next most common joint involved in hemophilia?

A. Shoulder
B. Elbow
C. Hip
D. Ankle

10 The finding below is classically associated with which disease?

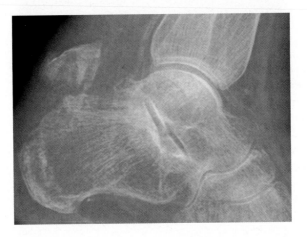

A. Hyperparathyroidism
B. Renal osteodystrophy
C. Diabetes mellitus
D. Osteomalacia

11a Which of the below statements is the most accurate internal standard for evaluating the MRI appearance of red marrow?

A. The T1-weighted signal of red marrow is greater than skeletal muscle or intervertebral discs.
B. The T1-weighted signal of red marrow is less than skeletal muscle or intervertebral discs.
C. The T2-weighted signal of red marrow is greater than skeletal muscle or intervertebral discs.
D. The T2-weighted signal of red marrow is less than skeletal muscle or intervertebral discs.

11b Which portion of the bone converts red marrow to yellow marrow last?

    A. Epiphysis
    B. Apophysis
    C. Metaphysis
    D. Diaphysis

11c Which of the following is the most characteristic imaging appearance of mass-like extramedullary hematopoiesis?

    A. Homogeneous nonfatty soft tissue masses in the appendicular skeleton
    B. Homogeneous nonfatty soft tissue masses in the axial skeleton
    C. Heterogeneously fatty soft tissue masses in the appendicular skeleton
    D. Heterogeneously fatty soft tissue masses in the axial skeleton

12a A 34-year-old male presents with back and pelvic pain. What is the most likely cause of the bone marrow signal pattern?

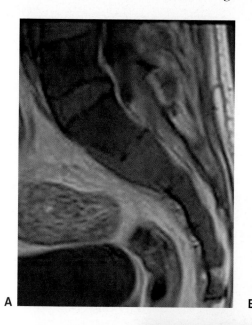
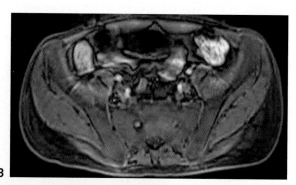
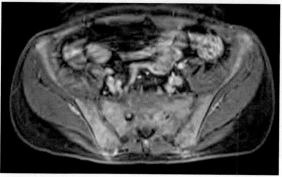

A. Sagittal T1 weighted **B.** Axial T1 weighted fat saturated **C.** Axial T1 weighted fat saturated postcontrast

    A. Marrow reconversion
    B. Sickle cell anemia
    C. Aplastic anemia
    D. Malignancy

12b A 21-year-old male presents with hip and pelvic pain. What is the most likely cause of the bone marrow signal pattern?

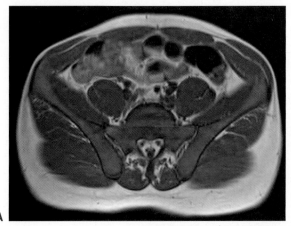 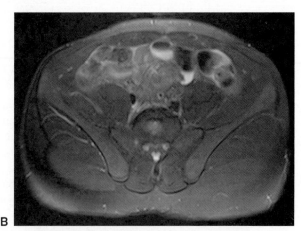

A. Axial T1 weighted **B.** Axial T2 weighted fat saturated

A. Marrow reconversion
B. Sickle cell anemia
C. Aplastic anemia
D. Malignancy

12c A 20-year-old college athlete presents with right shoulder pain after a recent increase in training before the beginning of the season. What is the most likely cause of the bone marrow signal pattern?

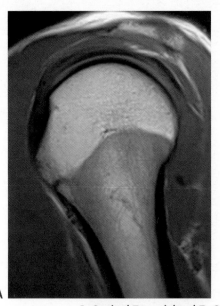 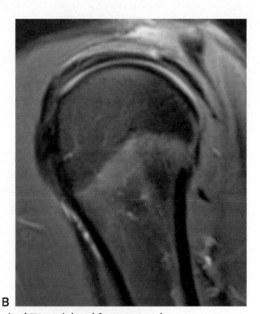

A. Sagittal T1 weighted **B.** Sagittal T2 weighted fat saturated

A. Marrow reconversion
B. Sickle cell anemia
C. Aplastic anemia
D. Malignancy

13 Which of the following diseases is depicted in the following radiograph?

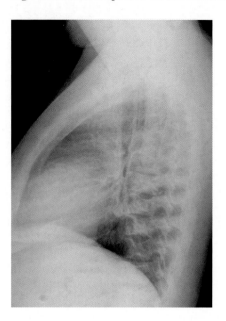

A. Sickle cell disease
B. Extramedullary hematopoiesis
C. Hemophilia
D. Osteoporosis

ANSWERS AND EXPLANATIONS

1   **Answer D.**   Looser zones represent pseudofractures. In the femur, they are characteristically noted inferior to the lesser trochanter on the medial side of the subtrochanteric region of the femur. They represent focal deposition of uncalcified osteoid, seen as an ill-defined horizontal linear lucency in the cortex that does not span the complete diameter of the bone. They may have sclerosis parallel to the margins. These are often bilaterally symmetric. In addition to the femur, they may also be seen in the pubic rami, axillary margin of the scapula, ribs, and the proximal ulna.

References: Manaster BJ, Roberts CC, Petersilge CA, et al. *Diagnostic Imaging: Musculoskeletal: Non-Traumatic Disease*. Manitoba, Canada: Amirsys; 2010:11:14–17.
Weissman BN. *Imaging of Arthritis and Metabolic Bone Disease*. Philadelphia, PA: Saunders; 2009:662.

2a   **Answer B.**   The shoulder radiograph depicts subchondral resorption of the distal clavicle and possible subtendinous resorption of the greater tuberosity at the supraspinatus tendon insertion. The knee radiograph demonstrates subtle subperiosteal resorption of the medial surface of the tibial metaphysis. These findings are typical of hyperparathyroidism.

References: Manaster BJ, Roberts CC, Petersilge CA, et al. *Diagnostic Imaging: Musculoskeletal: Non-Traumatic Disease*. Manitoba, Canada: Amirsys; 2010:11:8–13.
Weissman BN. *Imaging of Arthritis and Metabolic Bone Disease*. Philadelphia, PA: Saunders; 2009:642–649.

2b   **Answer D.**   All of the findings described are consistent with hyperparathyroidism; however, the earliest finding radiographically is subperiosteal resorption of the radial surface of the second and third digit middle phalanx of the hand. Radiographic findings of hyperparathyroidism include osteoporosis, subperiosteal resorption, subchondral resorption, subtendinous and subligamentous resorption, physeal resorption, acroosteolysis, brown tumors, soft tissue calcifications, and chondrocalcinosis.

References: Manaster BJ, Roberts CC, Petersilge CA, et al. *Diagnostic Imaging: Musculoskeletal: Non-Traumatic Disease*. Manitoba, Canada: Amirsys; 2010:11:8–13.
Weissman BN. *Imaging of Arthritis and Metabolic Bone Disease*. Philadelphia, PA: Saunders; 2009:642–649.

2c   **Answer A.**   75% to 85% of cases of primary hyperparathyroidism are attributed to a parathyroid adenoma. 10% to 20% are due to parathyroid hyperplasia, and 1% to 5% are due to a parathyroid carcinoma.

References: Manaster BJ, Roberts CC, Petersilge CA, et al. *Diagnostic Imaging: Musculoskeletal: Non-Traumatic Disease*. Manitoba, Canada: Amirsys; 2010:11:8–13.
Weissman BN. *Imaging of Arthritis and Metabolic Bone Disease*. Philadelphia, PA: Saunders; 2009:642–649.

3   **Answer B.**   The thickened heel pad is considered classic for acromegaly. A heel pad is considered thickened if it is >2.3 cm in a male and 2.15 cm in a female. Other findings noted in acromegaly include widened joint and disc spaces, cranial thickening, osteophytosis, thickened diaphysis of the long bones, spade-like terminal tufts of the distal phalanges, and degenerative arthropathy.

Reference: Manaster BJ, Roberts CC, Petersilge CA, et al. *Diagnostic Imaging: Musculoskeletal: Non-Traumatic Disease*. Manitoba, Canada: Amirsys; 2010:11:36–37.

4a **Answer B.**   The image depicts cortical hypertrophy with a cortical break on the lateral femoral cortex with an associated transverse fracture arising from the lateral femoral cortex. Given the patient is a 75-year-old female with osteoporosis, the finding is most consistent with a fracture associated with bisphosphonate therapy. These can be seen in the setting of a low-velocity trauma but may occur in the absence of trauma. Looser zones and stress fractures are seen within the medial femoral cortex.

Reference: Manaster BJ, Roberts CC, Petersilge CA, et al. *Diagnostic Imaging: Musculoskeletal: Non-Traumatic Disease*. Manitoba, Canada: Amirsys; 2010:12:10.

4b **Answer A.**   The most appropriate next step is to screen the contralateral femur/hip because these fractures may be bilateral, even in the absence of pain on the contralateral side.

Reference: Manaster BJ, Roberts CC, Petersilge CA, et al. *Diagnostic Imaging: Musculoskeletal: Non-Traumatic Disease*. Manitoba, Canada: Amirsys; 2010:12:10.

4c **Answer C.**   The best imaging test used to diagnose osteoporosis is a DEXA scan. In conjunction with the DEXA scan, radiographs of the AP lumbar spine, hips, and nondominant forearm are correlated; however, a skeletal survey alone is insufficient in diagnosing osteoporosis. An MRI of the lumbar spine and sacrum currently has no accepted role in the diagnosis of osteoporosis.

Reference: Manaster BJ, Roberts CC, Petersilge CA, et al. *Diagnostic Imaging: Musculoskeletal: Non-Traumatic Disease*. Manitoba, Canada: Amirsys; 2010:11:28–31.

5 **Answer C.**   Soft tissue calcifications in the setting of renal osteodystrophy typically present in periarticular locations, such as the hips and shoulders. The calcifications are the result of calcium hydroxyapatite crystal deposition. These crystals may cause pressure erosions on the adjacent bone. They tend to increase in severity and number when the patient is on dialysis. Calcium pyrophosphate may also occur in the setting of renal osteodystrophy, but this presents as chondrocalcinosis and not soft tissue calcifications. Uric acid, or sodium urate, crystals are associated with gout. Findings associated with secondary hyperparathyroidism, osteomalacia, osteoporosis, and neostosis may also be seen in the setting of renal osteodystrophy.

References: Manaster BJ, Roberts CC, Petersilge CA, et al. *Diagnostic Imaging: Musculoskeletal: Non-Traumatic Disease*. Manitoba, Canada: Amirsys; 2010:11:18–23.
Weissman BN. *Imaging of Arthritis and Metabolic Bone Disease*. Philadelphia, PA: Saunders; 2009:649–655.

6 **Answer D.**   Thyroid acropachy typically occurs after treatment is initiated in a patient with Graves disease. This disease may occur years after treatment began. Periosteal new bone formation has a lacy appearance, is asymmetric in distribution, and most commonly affects the upper extremities. The most common location is the metacarpals. It typically involves the radial aspect of the first through fourth metacarpals and the ulnar aspect of the fifth metacarpal.

Reference: Manaster BJ, Roberts CC, Petersilge CA, et al. *Diagnostic Imaging: Musculoskeletal: Non-Traumatic Disease*. Manitoba, Canada: Amirsys; 2010:11:40–41.

7 **Answer A.**   In myelofibrosis, the normal intramedullary fat is replaced by fibrosis; therefore, the T1-weighted signal, which in normal patients is greater than the intervertebral discs and muscle, becomes hypointense in comparison with these same structures. In the same manner, due to the relative absence of intramedullary fat, the opposed-phase images do not show the drop in signal compared to the in-phase images seen characteristically due to fat. In myelofibrosis, the intramedullary signal remains low on both the T2-weighted and STIR sequences. Additionally, the marrow signal does not enhance, which helps distinguish myelofibrosis from diffuse marrow replacement by tumor.

Reference: Manaster BJ, Roberts CC, Petersilge CA, et al. *Diagnostic Imaging: Musculoskeletal: Non-Traumatic Disease*. Manitoba, Canada: Amirsys; 2010:6:20–21.

8 **Answer C.**   Thalassemia leads to expansion of the medullary cavity of bones. This expansion is the result of anemia, hemosiderin deposition, and fibrosis. In the long tubular bones, this expansion is seen as squaring of the bones and loss of the normal tubulation. Diffuse osteopenia and extramedullary hematopoiesis may also be seen. In the skull, the diploic space is widened and the trabeculae are thickened. These changes cause the characteristic "hair-on-end" appearance. In the spine, there is a relative paucity of horizontal trabeculae. The trabeculae present are thickened, leading to a striated appearance. On MRI, the marrow may be low in signal on both T1- and T2-weighted MR sequences, while the hemosiderin deposition in the marrow may demonstrate blooming on a GRE sequence.

Reference: Manaster BJ, Roberts CC, Petersilge CA, et al. *Diagnostic Imaging: Musculoskeletal: Non-Traumatic Disease*. Manitoba, Canada: Amirsys; 2010:6:16–19.

9a **Answer D.**   The image depicts the typical findings of hemophilia. The findings include unilateral overgrowth of the right femur distal epiphysis and metaphysis, osteopenia, widening of the intercondylar notch, and cartilage destruction depicted by joint space loss in the medial and lateral compartments of the knee. The diaphysis of the femur is gracile; however, it is only partially visualized on the image. These findings are the result of recurrent bleeding into the joint, leading to synovitis and hyperemia, which in turn creates the characteristic findings. The differential diagnosis would include juvenile idiopathic arthritis (JIA), tuberculosis arthritis, and pigmented villonodular synovitis (PVNS). JIA may look very similar to hemophilia radiographically and also occurs in the skeletally immature; therefore, history and lab tests may be helpful to distinguish the two. PVNS is less common in the skeletally immature patient, and when it does occur, it does not result in the same degree of overgrowth of the epiphysis and metaphysis that hemophilia does. Tuberculosis arthritis leads to slower cartilage destruction and erosion formation than a pyogenic infection caused by *S. aureus*; therefore, it has a radiographic appearance similar to hemophilia. Disuse osteopenia and chondrocalcinosis would not result in the characteristic findings of hemophilia.

References: Manaster BJ, Roberts CC, Petersilge CA, et al. *Diagnostic Imaging: Musculoskeletal: Non-Traumatic Disease*. Manitoba, Canada: Amirsys; 2010:6:22–27.
Weissman BN. *Imaging of Arthritis and Metabolic Bone Disease*. Philadelphia, PA: Saunders; 2009:447–449.

9b **Answer B.**   The most common joint involved in hemophilia is the knee followed in order by the elbow, ankle, hip, and shoulder. In the elbow, the classic finding is overgrowth of the radial head.

References: Manaster BJ, Roberts CC, Petersilge CA, et al. *Diagnostic Imaging: Musculoskeletal: Non-Traumatic Disease*. Manitoba, Canada: Amirsys; 2010:6:22–27.
Weissman BN. *Imaging of Arthritis and Metabolic Bone Disease*. Philadelphia, PA: Saunders; 2009:447–449.

10 **Answer C.**   The image demonstrates a calcaneal insufficiency avulsion (CIA) fracture, which is thought to be specific for diabetes. This is seen as elevation of the posterior tubercle by the Achilles tendon.

References: Manaster BJ, Roberts CC, Petersilge CA, et al. *Diagnostic Imaging: Musculoskeletal: Non-Traumatic Disease*. Manitoba, Canada: Amirsys; 2010:6:28–33.
Weissman BN. *Imaging of Arthritis and Metabolic Bone Disease*. Philadelphia, PA: Saunders; 2009:653–654.

11a Answer A.   The internal standard for characterizing red marrow on MRI is that the normal red marrow is higher in T1-weighted signal in comparison to skeletal muscle or intervertebral discs. Red marrow comprises ~40% fat; thus, it has a greater signal intensity when compared to muscle or intervertebral discs. There is no reliable T2-weighted internal standard for evaluating red marrow.

Reference: Manaster BJ, Roberts CC, Petersilge CA, et al. *Diagnostic Imaging: Musculoskeletal: Non-Traumatic Disease.* Manitoba, Canada: Amirsys; 2010:9:2–5.

11b Answer C.   Red marrow converts to yellow marrow in the following order: epiphysis and apophysis, diaphysis, and finally the metaphysis. The conversion begins in the distal extremities and progresses proximally. By 20 to 25 years of age, the appendicular skeleton is mostly fatty marrow; the exception is the proximal metaphysis of the humerus and femur, which may retain red marrow in the normal patient.

Reference: Manaster BJ, Roberts CC, Petersilge CA, et al. *Diagnostic Imaging: Musculoskeletal: Non-Traumatic Disease.* Manitoba, Canada: Amirsys; 2010:9:2–5.

11c Answer D.   Masses in extramedullary hematopoiesis are characteristically well defined, multiple, and located in the axial skeleton and contain macroscopic internal fat.

References: Ginzel AW, Kransdorf MJ, Peterson JJ, et al. Mass-like extramedullary hematopoiesis: imaging features. *Skeletal Radiol.* 2012;41(8):911–916.
Resnick D, Kang HS, Pretterklieber ML. *Internal Derangements of Joints.* 2nd ed. Philadelphia, PA: Saunders; 2007:244.

12a Answer D.   The sagittal T1 image demonstrates the bone marrow signal to be higher than the intervertebral disc, consistent with red marrow. The axial images demonstrate diffuse enhancement of the bone marrow, consistent with malignancy. This case is an example of leukemia.

Reference: Manaster BJ, Roberts CC, Petersilge CA, et al. *Diagnostic Imaging: Musculoskeletal: Non-Traumatic Disease.* Manitoba, Canada: Amirsys; 2010:9:6–17.

12b Answer B.   This case demonstrates diffuse red marrow reconversion of the entirety of the visualized pelvis and sacrum. Given the options provided, this appearance is most consistent with sickle cell disease.

Reference: Manaster BJ, Roberts CC, Petersilge CA, et al. *Diagnostic Imaging: Musculoskeletal: Non-Traumatic Disease.* Manitoba, Canada: Amirsys; 2010:9:6–11.

12c Answer A.   The metaphysis of the humerus demonstrates T1-weighted signal higher than the adjacent muscle. This is consistent with red marrow. This may be interpreted as within normal limits for the patient's age or could be considered red marrow reconversion due to a need for increased red marrow resulting from increased training. Red marrow reconversion progresses in the reverse order as seen for red-to-yellow marrow conversion, meaning the axial skeleton converts first followed by the metaphysis, diaphysis, and then the epiphysis and apophysis of the appendicular skeleton. The differential diagnosis for increased red marrow includes red marrow reconversion, red marrow repopulation in conditions such as sickle cell disease and thalassemia, red marrow stimulation from medications, rebound from chemotherapy, marrow deposition diseases, myelofibrosis, and tumors. Other than red marrow reconversion, these additional diseases would be expected to have more marrow reconversion than what is seen in this case. Given the provided history, however, the most likely cause is marrow reconversion associated with increased training. Aplastic anemia results in decreased red marrow. Diagnosis of malignancy involving the marrow is aided by contrast-enhanced studies.

Reference: Manaster BJ, Roberts CC, Petersilge CA, et al. *Diagnostic Imaging: Musculoskeletal: Non-Traumatic Disease.* Manitoba, Canada: Amirsys; 2010:9:6–11.

13 **Answer A.** Sickle cell disease is a hemolytic anemia that manifests in a myriad of ways. In this patient, cardiac enlargement from chronic anemia is present. The fish-vertebra sign, which is present, is a biconcave vertebral body deformity characteristically occurring as a result of squared-off depression of the vertebral end plates and compression by adjacent intervertebral discs. In the sickle cell patient, the radiologist should be alert for gallstones, osteonecrosis, sequelae of marrow expansion, and pneumonia.

Reference: Ejindu VC, Hine AL, Mashayekhi M, et al. Musculoskeletal manifestations of sickle cell disease. *Radiographics.* 2007;27:1005–1021.

8

Arthropathy

1   A 72-year-old female presented with the following radiograph 2 years after
surgery. What is the cause of the imaged process?

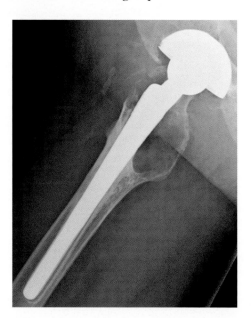

A. Normal wear
B. Hemophilia
C. An infectious process
D. A histiocytic response

2   Which of the following connective tissue disorders has soft tissue calcifications
as a prominent manifestation of the disease on radiographs?

A. Rheumatoid arthritis
B. Polymyositis
C. Systemic lupus erythematosus
D. Calcium pyrophosphate dihydrate (CPPD) arthropathy

3a A patient with a history of an inflammatory arthropathy presents for imaging. The provided radiographs demonstrate which of the following findings?

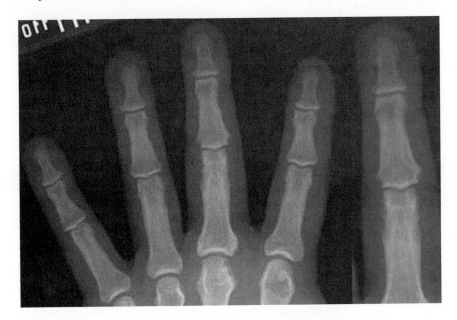

A. Acroosteolysis
B. Sausage digit
C. Gouty tophi
D. Periarticular osteopenia
E. Central "gull wing" erosions

3b Based on the images provided, what is the most likely diagnosis?

A. Rheumatoid arthritis
B. Tophaceous gout
C. Scleroderma
D. Erosive osteoarthritis
E. Psoriatic arthritis

4 A 15-year-old male presents with the images of the feet below. In this disease, what location most commonly undergoes ankylosis?

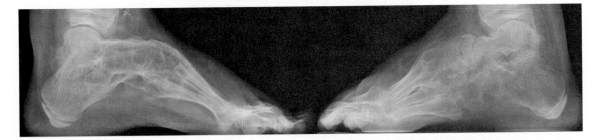

A. Tarsal bones
B. Carpal bones
C. Hips
D. Lumbar spine

5   What typical findings of calcium pyrophosphate dihydrate (CPPD) arthropathy are noted in the image below?

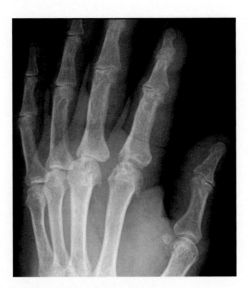

   A. Joint space narrowing and marginal erosions
   B. Bone demineralization and central erosions
   C. Large subchondral cysts and hooked osteophytes
   D. Enthesophytes and eburnation

6   What disease process is depicted in the images below?

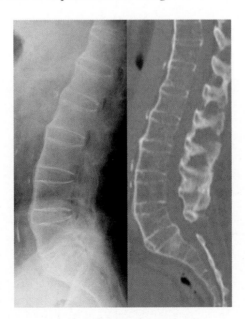

   A. Ankylosing spondylitis
   B. Diffuse idiopathic skeletal hyperostosis
   C. Psoriatic arthritis
   D. Reactive arthritis

7 The imaged metabolic disease manifests as an arthropathy characterized by excessive intra-articular and periarticular deposition of what substance?

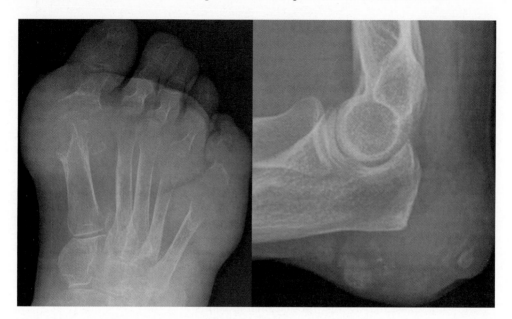

A. Calcium pyrophosphate dihydrate crystals
B. Hemosiderin
C. Monosodium urate crystals
D. B2 microglobulin

8 Bilateral hand and wrist radiographs are pictured below. What additional imaging finding, outside of the hands and wrists, may also be seen in this same disease process?

- soft tissue
  calcifications
- acro-osteolysis

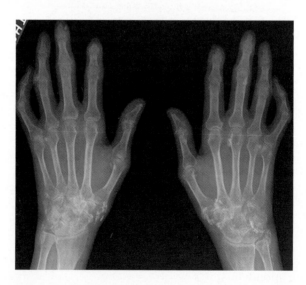

A. Esophagram demonstrating achalasia
B. High-resolution chest CT revealing changes of lymphangioleiomyomatosis
C. AP pelvis showing bilaterally symmetric sacroiliitis
D. Small bowel follow-through showing dilated small bowel with closely spaced, thin folds

9 Axial T1-weighted and sagittal T2-weighted fat-saturated MR images
   demonstrate a mass-like focus within the anterior joint space of the knee. Of
   the choices below, which is the most likely diagnosis?

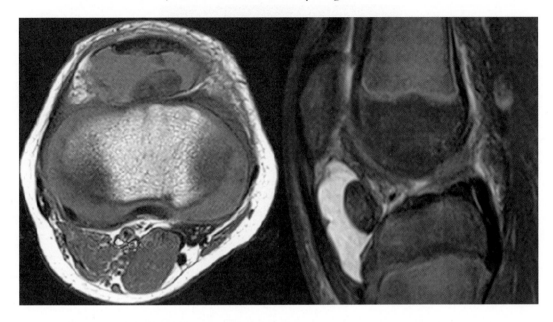

A. Amyloidosis
B. Pigmented villonodular synovitis
C. Osteochondromatosis
D. Rheumatoid arthritis

10 An 81-year-old male presents with left hip pain. A mass is noted in the
    expected location of the iliopsoas bursa on the images below. If aspiration of
    this mass is performed, what would the aspirate most likely resemble?

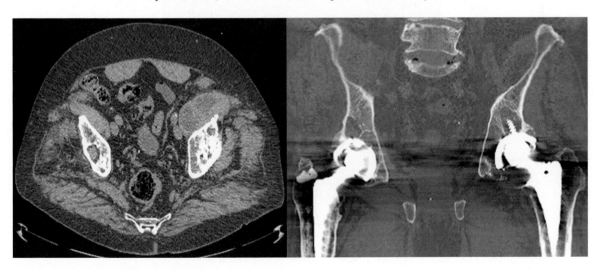

A. Gelatinous material
B. Purulent material
C. Bloody material
D. Serous material

11 A hand radiograph of a patient with rheumatoid arthritis is provided. Which of the following correctly describes the early erosions seen in this disease process?

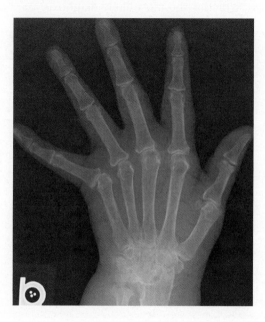

A. Periarticular at the interphalangeal joints and first carpometacarpal joint of the hand
B. Juxta-articular at the first metatarsophalangeal joint in the foot
C. Marginal at the ulnar styloid process and carpal bones of the wrist
D. Central at the metacarpophalangeal joints of the hands

12 The CT image of the pelvis below is most characteristic of which process?

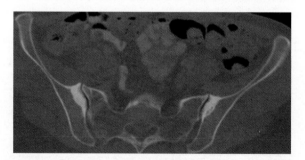

A. Osteitis condensans ilii
B. Ankylosing spondylitis
C. Sacroiliac joint septic arthritis
D. Reactive arthritis
E. Enteropathic sacroiliitis

13 What is the characteristic distribution of osteoarthritis?

A. Metacarpophalangeal joints and distal radioulnar joints
B. Proximal interphalangeal and pisotriquetral joints
C. Intercarpal and index finger metacarpophalangeal joints
D. Distal interphalangeal and thumb carpometacarpal joints

14 A 35-year-old female presents with the following radiographs of the right hand and wrist. What is the most likely diagnosis?

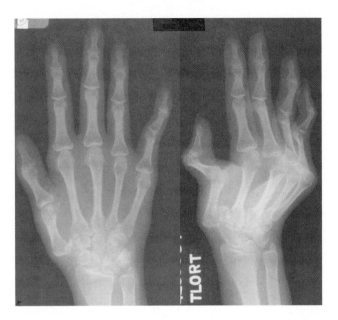

    A. Progressive systemic sclerosis
    B. Systemic lupus erythematosus
    C. Psoriatic arthritis
    D. Calcium pyrophosphate dihydrate (CPPD) arthropathy

15 A 55-year-old patient presents with the following radiograph of the lumbar spine. What is the most likely diagnosis?

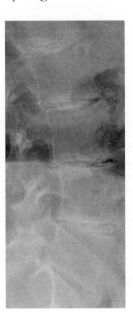

    A. Degenerative disc disease
    B. Hemochromatosis
    C. Ochronosis
    D. Spondylitis

16   The image of the hand below demonstrates acroosteolysis. Which disease process has imaging findings including acroosteolysis?

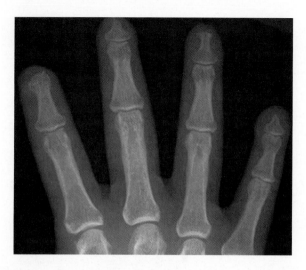

A. Mixed connective tissue disease
B. Calcium pyrophosphate dihydrate (CPPD) arthropathy
C. Rheumatoid arthritis
D. Ankylosing spondylitis

17   A radiograph of the index, middle, and ring fingers is presented. Asymmetric, nonerosive soft tissue swelling around the index finger proximal interphalangeal joint in a patient with underlying osteophytosis is characteristic of what deformity?

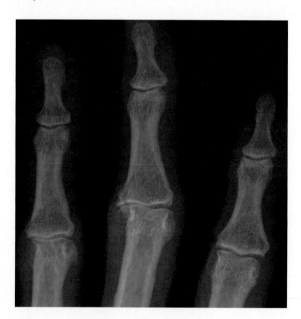

A. Boutonnière deformity
B. Mallet finger
C. Sausage finger
D. Bouchard node

18 The numerous joint and synovial findings seen in the lateral radiograph of the knee are most consistent with which pathology?

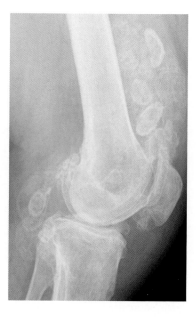

    A. Synovial osteochondromatosis
    B. Osteoarthritis
    C. Myositis ossificans
    D. Pigmented villonodular synovitis

19 A 35-year-old female presents with the following radiograph of the sacroiliac joints. Her radiograph of the lumbar spine, not presented, demonstrates thin, vertical syndesmophytes. What is the most likely diagnosis?

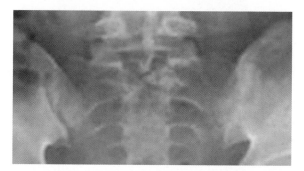

    A. Psoriatic arthritis
    B. Crohn disease
    C. Reactive arthritis
    D. Septic arthritis

20a Which of the following is a component of the classic triad of symptoms in reactive arthritis?

    A. Cholecystitis
    B. Colitis
    C. Skin calcifications
    D. Urethritis

20b Which of the following genitourinary infections is classically associated with reactive arthritis?

A. *Chlamydia trachomatis*
B. *Treponema pallidum*
C. *Neisseria gonorrhoeae*
D. *Trichomonas vaginalis*

21 In seronegative spondyloarthropathies, where do erosions and sclerosis typically present in the sacroiliac joints?

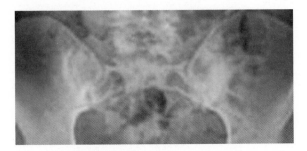

A. Sacral side of the inferior sacroiliac joint
B. Iliac side of the inferior sacroiliac joint
C. Sacral side of the superior sacroiliac joint
D. Iliac side of the superior sacroiliac joint

22 The skin calcifications in the image below are typical of which disease process?

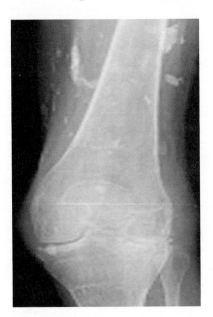

A. Calcium pyrophosphate dihydrate (CPPD) arthropathy
B. Dermatomyositis
C. Psoriatic arthritis
D. Systemic lupus erythematosus

23 Calcium pyrophosphate dihydrate (CPPD) deposition arthropathy of the hands and wrists presents with bilaterally symmetric subchondral cysts, beak-like osteophytes, and chondrocalcinosis in a proximal distribution. These findings are similar to which other arthropathy?

    A. Reactive arthritis
    B. Rheumatoid arthritis
    C. Hemochromatosis
    D. Gout

24 The posterior lumbar facets are synovial-lined joints. Which part of the lumbar facet joint first shows changes of degeneration?

    A. Inferior articulating process
    B. Spinous process
    C. Ligamentum flavum
    D. Superior articulating process

25 Radiographs of the lumbar spine, 3 years prior and current, are presented for evaluation. Which of the following complications has occurred in the interval?

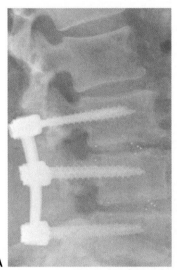 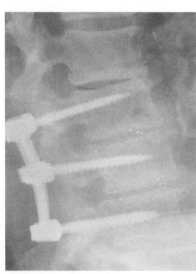

A. 3 years prior **B.** Current

    A. Hardware fracture
    B. Degenerative disc disease
    C. Compression fracture
    D. Spondylolysis

26 Which of the following may occur in connective tissue disease?

    A. Tumoral calcinosis
    B. Calcific tendonitis
    C. Hydroxyapatite deposition
    D. Calcinosis circumscripta

27 Which of the following arthropathies manifests as cartilage loss in the weight-bearing portions of a joint, bone proliferation, and subchondral cyst formation?

    A. Psoriatic arthritis
    B. Osteoarthritis
    C. Reactive arthritis
    D. Rheumatoid arthritis

28 A thoracic spine radiograph is presented below, what is the most likely diagnosis?

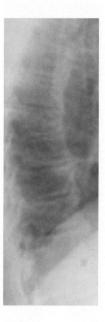

    A. Rheumatoid arthritis
    B. Psoriatic arthritis
    C. Diffuse idiopathic skeletal hyperostosis
    D. Ankylosing spondylitis

29 The abnormally increased subchondral bone mineral density in this patient is most likely the result of which process?

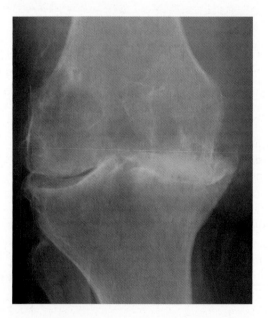

    A. Fluorosis
    B. Osteoarthritis
    C. Paget disease
    D. Renal osteodystrophy

30a What arthropathy is noted involving the thumb carpometacarpal joint in the radiographs shown below?

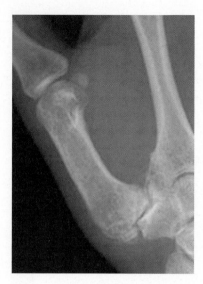

    A. Reactive arthritis
    B. Rheumatoid arthritis
    C. Osteoarthritis
    D. Ankylosing spondylitis

30b What are the bony excrescences that extend from the trapezium in this patient?
    A. Osteophytes
    B. Enthesophytes
    C. Syndesmophytes
    D. Erosions

31 What inflammatory arthropathy finding is most pronounced in the images below?

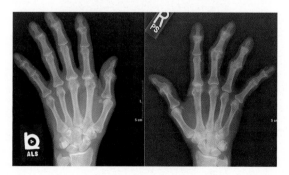

    A. Central erosions
    B. Periarticular osteopenia
    C. Periostitis
    D. Subchondral cysts

32 Periostitis is seen in which of the following arthropathies?
    A. Psoriatic arthritis
    B. Rheumatoid arthritis
    C. Gout
    D. Osteoarthritis

33   What is the direction of joint space narrowing in this patient?

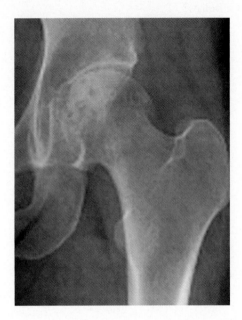

A. Superior
B. Posterior
C. Axial
D. Inferior

34   A 20-year-old male presents with the cervical spine radiograph below. The findings noted in the cervical spine most commonly occur at what level?

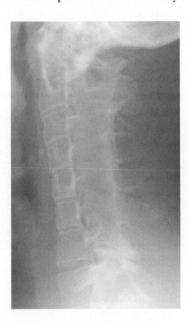

A. C1–C2
B. C2–C3
C. C4–C5
D. C5–C6

35 In this image of a medial compartment prosthesis, which of the following complications is present?

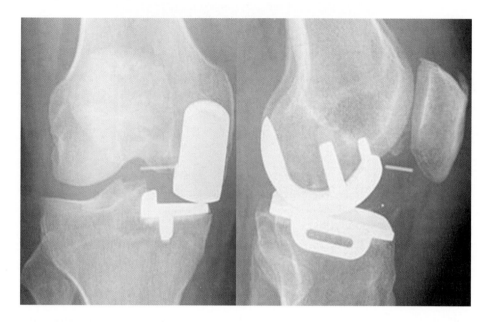

A. Hardware loosening
B. Infection
C. Spacer displacement
D. Fracture

36 Progressive great toe osteoarthritis consisting of osteophyte formation, joint space narrowing, and subchondral sclerosis can lead to what condition?

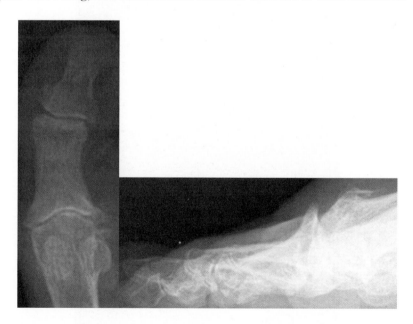

A. Hallux rigidus
B. Hallux valgus
C. Turf toe
D. Morton syndrome

37 What is the diagnosis based on the provided AP radiograph of the bilateral feet?

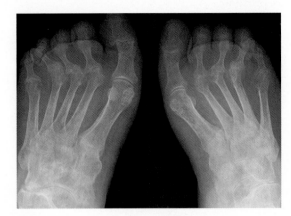

    A. Ankylosing spondylitis
    B. Psoriatic arthritis
    C. Osteoarthritis
    D. Rheumatoid arthritis
    E. Gout

38 What is the earliest radiographic manifestation of the arthropathy depicted in the hands and wrists below?

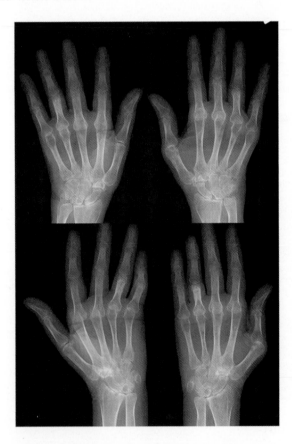

    A. Soft tissue swelling and juxta-articular osteoporosis
    B. Erosions of the ulnar styloid and metacarpal heads
    C. Radiocarpal and interphalangeal joint space narrowing
    D. Metacarpophalangeal joint subluxation

39   What is the most likely etiology of the findings at the L3–L4 level on the CT image below?

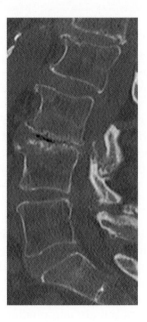

A. Ankylosing spondylitis
B. Degenerative disc disease
C. Discitis–osteomyelitis
D. Diffuse idiopathic skeletal hyperostosis

40   Which of the following radiographic findings is the most sensitive for the detection of arthroplasty loosening?

A. Any bone cement lucency
B. Change in the position of the hardware
C. Stress shielding
D. Polyethylene component wear

ANSWERS AND EXPLANATIONS

1   **Answer D.**   Particle disease is also known as aggressive granulomatosis. It is a histiocytic response of the bone to small polyethylene particles shed from the lining of the hardware. It causes localized osteolysis and may demonstrate a superiorly malpositioned femoral head component. The provided image demonstrates a large lucency around the femoral component of the arthroplasty, consistent with osteolysis. Treatment commonly requires revision. The collection around the hip can be distinguished clinically from infection by lack of night pain and fever, but hip aspiration may be required to confirm the diagnosis.

Reference: Garcia GM. *Musculoskeletal Radiology*. New York, NY: Thieme; 2010:66.

2   **Answer B.**   Connective tissue diseases that may have radiographic apparent soft tissue calcifications include scleroderma, dermatomyositis, and polymyositis. Calcification in scleroderma and polymyositis may not be distinguishable from each other, but scleroderma will usually have other soft tissue resorptive changes and skin tightening to aid in the diagnosis. Soft tissue calcifications may be present but are not a hallmark of SLE or rheumatoid arthritis. Hydroxyapatite crystal deposition disease has calcifications associated with the joints and tendons. Polymyositis is a rare autoimmune disorder of unknown cause characterized by inflammation and degeneration of muscle. The characteristic late finding on radiographs is widespread soft tissue calcification, commonly seen in the intermuscular fascial planes. The diagnosis is based on a typical clinical presentation, elevated serum skeletal muscle enzymes, electromyography findings, and an abnormal muscle biopsy. In the most common clinical form of polymyositis, there is gradually increasing proximal limb weakness with later involvement of the laryngeal and pharyngeal muscles. Joint manifestations, which can be similar to SLE or rheumatoid arthritis, may be seen in 20% to 50% of patients.

References: Chew FS. *Musculoskeletal Imaging: The Core Curriculum Series*. Philadelphia, PA: Lippincott Williams & Wilkins; 2003:361.
Schulze M, Kötter I, Ernemann U, et al. MRI findings in inflammatory muscle diseases and their noninflammatory mimics. *AJR Am J Roentgenol*. 2009;192(6):1708–1716.

3a   **Answer B.**   Radiographs demonstrate fusiform soft tissue swelling about the long finger, a finding referred to as the sausage digit. The central "gull wing" erosion characteristic of erosive osteoarthritis is not present in this case. Acroosteolysis, periarticular osteopenia, and gouty tophi are also absent in this case.

Reference: Brower AC, Flemming DJ. *Arthritis in Black and White*. 3rd ed. Philadelphia, PA: Saunders; 2012:200–203.

3b   **Answer E.**   The provided images also demonstrate marginal erosions of the middle phalanx and fluffy periosteal new bone formation. Overall, the constellation of findings makes psoriatic arthritis the most likely diagnosis. The "sausage digit" is commonly associated with psoriatic arthritis; however, one must carefully consider the clinical context and associated findings, as cellulitis could appear similar. The erosions of psoriatic arthritis initially occur at the margins of joints, but may progress ultimately to involve the central bone and result in the classic "pencil in cup" deformity. Bone mineral density is usually preserved in psoriatic arthritis, in contrast to the prominent periarticular osteopenia seen with rheumatoid arthritis. Bone proliferation is a prominent feature of psoriatic arthritis and may occur along the shaft of a bone, adjacent to erosions, or at tendinous or ligamentous insertions. Psoriatic arthritis is seen in only 5% of individuals afflicted with skin disease; however, in rare instances, radiographic findings may be the first manifestation of disease.

Reference: Brower AC, Flemming DJ. *Arthritis in Black and White*. 3rd ed. Philadelphia, PA: Saunders; 2012:200–203.

4   Answer B.   The carpal bones are the most frequent site of ankylosis in the setting of juvenile idiopathic arthritis (JIA). Another common location is the cervical spine where there is ankylosis of the apophyseal joints leading to a decrease in size of the adjoining vertebral bodies. Ankylosis is considered a late finding in the disease progression.

References: Manaster BJ, Roberts CC, Petersilge CA, et al. *Diagnostic Imaging: Musculoskeletal: Non-Traumatic Disease*. Philadelphia, PA: Amirsys; 2010;1:40–45.
Weissman BN. *Imaging of Arthritis and Metabolic Bone Disease*. Philadelphia, PA: Saunders; 2009:428–437.

5   Answer C.   Calcium pyrophosphate dihydrate crystal deposition disease is a polyarticular arthritis as a result of crystal deposition. The crystals form in the cartilage, joint capsule, ligaments, tendons, and discs. Deposition in the hyaline articular cartilage of a joint results in structural damage. The distribution of joint involvement is proximal but can be very similar to the distribution of osteoarthritis. The radiocarpal joint is involved, which can classically result in scapholunate ligament tear, scapholunate dissociation, and eventually scapholunate advanced collapse (SLAC wrist). Hook-like or drooping osteophytes are a distinctive feature of the hand, most commonly seen arising from the second and third metacarpal heads. There may be associated subchondral cysts. In the knee, the patellofemoral compartment is classically involved out of proportion to the femorotibial compartments. Chondrocalcinosis may be radiographically evident in the menisci of the knee as well. The glenohumeral joint, elbow, ankle, and foot can be involved. Chondrocalcinosis is not always present.

Reference: Chew FS. *Musculoskeletal Imaging: The Core Curriculum Series*. Philadelphia, PA: Lippincott Williams & Wilkins; 2003:389–391.

6   Answer A.   Ankylosing spondylitis is an idiopathic inflammatory process predominantly in the sacroiliac joints and the spine. Typically, the disease ascends from the sacroiliac joints. The sacroiliitis can begin asymmetrically or unilaterally, but eventually becomes bilaterally symmetric. Initially, osteitis develops at the anterior corner of the vertebral bodies, manifesting as "shiny corners." The spine develops thin, vertical syndesmophytes, which develop within the outer fibers of the annulus fibrosus. Over time, fusion of the spine, known as bamboo spine, occurs, making the spine susceptible to three-column fractures/injuries. The disease is associated with HLA-B27. It affects <1% of the population.

Reference: Chew FS. *Musculoskeletal Imaging: The Core Curriculum Series*. Philadelphia, PA: Lippincott Williams & Wilkins; 2003:363–366.

7   Answer C.   Gout is associated with intra-articular and periarticular deposition of monosodium urate crystals. This results in an acute inflammatory and chronic granulomatous response, producing soft tissue swelling and tophi, with well-defined periarticular erosions with "overhanging" edges. The first metatarsophalangeal joint is most commonly involved. The arthropathy is commonly asymmetric and polyarticular and may be primary or due to conditions causing increase cell turnover. Joint spaces are preserved until late in the disease process. Calcium pyrophosphate dihydrate (CPPD) deposition–related arthropathy is known as pseudogout. Excessive intra-articular hemosiderin deposition can be seen in hemophilia and pigmented villonodular synovitis (PVNS). Intra-articular B2 microglobulin deposition is seen in the setting of amyloidosis.

Reference: Brower A, Flemming DJ. *Arthritis in Black and White*. Philadelphia, PA: Saunders; 2012:293–297.

8 Answer D.   Scleroderma is a progressive multisystem immunologic–mediated connective tissue disorder and small vessel vasculitis. There is variable involvement of the skin, GI tract, and lungs. Musculoskeletal radiographic features of scleroderma include soft tissue calcifications, soft tissue wasting, osteoporosis, and acroosteolysis. After the skin, the GI tract is the most frequently involved, with esophageal dysmotility and dilation, patulous gastroesophageal junction, dilated small bowel with closely spaced thin folds (hidebound bowel), and wide-mouthed sacculations. Some patients develop pulmonary fibrosis as a visceral complication. CREST syndrome is a variant of scleroderma with less severe visceral involvement, characterized by calcinosis, Raynaud phenomenon, esophageal dysmotility, and telangiectasias.

Reference: Brower AC, Flemming DJ. *Arthritis in Black and White*. 3rd ed. Philadelphia, PA: Saunders; 2012:352–353.

9 Answer B.   Pigmented villonodular synovitis is a benign neoplasm of the synovium with low MR signal intensity on T1- and T2-weighted images due to widespread hemosiderin deposition from repeated episodes of intra-articular hemorrhage. In the early stages, PVNS findings include joint effusion, juxta-articular erosions, and sparing of the joint space. In later stages, secondary osteoarthritis can develop due to a combination of repetitive bleeding and altered joint mechanics. Several entities can demonstrate synovial hypertrophy and bony erosions, but most have distinguishing characteristics. The lack of calcifications makes synovial osteochondromatosis much less likely. Low signal intensity on T2-weighted MR images may be seen with PVNS or amyloidosis, but PVNS is frequently a monoarticular process with a predilection for the knee, whereas amyloidosis is most often a systemic, polyarticular process. Any synovial joint may be involved. PVNS postresection recurrence rates may be as high as 50%, but malignancy in the setting of PVNS is rare.

Reference: Al-Nakshabandi NA, Ryan AG, Choudur H, et al. Pigmented villonodular synovitis. *Clin Radiol*. 59:414–420, 2004.

10 Answer A.   The lucency surrounding the right hip prosthesis hardware is the important finding, suggesting hardware loosening. In the hip, hardware loosening can lead to distention of the iliopsoas bursa. The bursa becomes filled with debris-laden macrophages, which are associated with particle disease. When the iliopsoas bursa or joint fluid is aspirated, the material is thick and gelatinous. If this were an iliopsoas abscess, it might be purulent. If this were a hematoma or pseudotumor from hemophilia, it might be bloody.

Reference: Manaster BJ, Roberts CC, Petersilge CA, et al. *Diagnostic Imaging: Musculoskeletal: Non-Traumatic Disease*. Philadelphia, PA: Amirsys; 2010;7:10–15.

11 Answer C.   Erosive change in rheumatoid arthritis is most typically characterized by marginal erosions. Early rheumatoid arthritis in the hand and wrist can present as small erosions in the metacarpal heads and proximal interphalangeal joints. The radial aspect of the proximal phalanges is at times involved as well. In the wrist, the early erosions of rheumatoid arthritis occur at the scaphoid waist, at the capitate, and at the fifth carpometacarpal articulation as well as the radial and ulnar styloids. Gout would typically have juxta-articular erosions about the great toe in the foot. While metacarpophalangeal joint involvement is frequently seen in rheumatoid arthritis, central erosions are more typical of erosive osteoarthritis.

Reference: Brower AC, Flemming DJ. *Arthritis in Black and White*. 3rd ed. Philadelphia, PA: Saunders; 2012:170–177.

12 **Answer A.** Benign, symmetric sclerosis predominantly on the iliac bone side of the sacroiliac joint is the hallmark of osteitis condensans ilii. It is rarely unilateral. The triangular-shaped sclerosis, with the apex pointed cephalad, is usually found in multiparous women but can also be seen in males. The patient may have low back symptoms, but the characteristic location should not be confused with sacroiliitis because the sacroiliac joints will generally be intact. No clear etiology has been determined. Bone scintigraphy may or may not show focal uptake at the site of sclerosis.

Reference: Manaster BJ, Roberts CC, Petersilge CA, et al. *Diagnostic Imaging: Musculoskeletal: Non-Traumatic Disease*. Philadelphia, PA: Amirsys; 2010;5:52–53.

13 **Answer D.** Osteoarthritis is the most common form of polyarticular arthritis, the prevalence of which increases with age. The classic distribution of hand osteoarthritis is the distal and proximal interphalangeal (IP) joints of the fingers, thumb carpometacarpal and IP joints, as well as the scaphoid–trapezoid–trapezium joint. Cartilage wear, as evidenced by fibrillation of the articular cartilage, is one of the earliest morphologic abnormalities resulting in asymmetric cartilage destruction. Subchondral cysts form through fissures in the worn cartilage. Bone hypertrophy is an adaptive healing response. This manifests as eburnation, also known as subchondral sclerosis, and osteophyte formation arising from the edges of the joint. Erosions and ankylosis should not be present. Soft tissue swelling is usually not prominent.

Reference: Chew FS, Mulcahy H, Ha AS. *Musculoskeletal Imaging: A Teaching File*. 3rd ed. Philadelphia, PA: Lippincott Williams & Wilkins; 2012:4.

14 **Answer B.** Systemic lupus erythematosus (lupus) is a multiorgan, autoimmune disease. The most frequent musculoskeletal finding is joint deformities without erosions. The deformities are typically reducible. Periarticular soft tissue swelling, osteoporosis, osteonecrosis, and tenosynovitis may also occur. Fixed deformities and secondary osteoarthritis may develop late in the disease. Musculoskeletal manifestation occurs in ~90% of patients with lupus.

References: Chew FS. *Musculoskeletal Imaging: The Core Curriculum Series*. Philadelphia, PA: Lippincott Williams and Wilkins; 2003:359.
Manaster BJ, Roberts CC, Petersilge CA, et al. *Diagnostic Imaging: Musculoskeletal: Non-Traumatic Disease*. Philadelphia, PA: Amirsys; 2010;6:58–61.

15 **Answer C.** Ochronosis is caused by the accumulation of homogentisic acid in connective tissues. The name comes from the yellowish, ocher-like, discoloration of the tissue under microscopy. The radiologic findings result from the accumulation of pigment deposits in the joints of the axial and peripheral skeleton. The spine findings are typified by osteopenia, disc space narrowing, calcifications, and the relative absence of significant osteophytosis in the thoracic and cervical spine. Loss of the normal lumbar lordosis, vacuum disc phenomenon, and disc calcifications that primarily involve the annulus fibrosus are additional findings. Marginal bridging intervertebral osteophytes, resembling the syndesmophytes in ankylosing spondylitis, are seen with long-standing disease. The disease involvement in the knees, glenohumeral joints, and hips may be indistinguishable from degenerative osteoarthritis; however, the young age of the patient may raise the suspicion for an alternate diagnosis to osteoarthritis. In the hands, the distal interphalangeal joint and thumb carpometacarpal joints may be involved.

Reference: Baeva M, Bueno A, Dhimes P. AIRP best cases in radiologic-pathologic correlation: ochronosis. *Radiographics*. 2011;31(4):1163–1167.

16   Answer A.   The term mixed connective tissue disease, also known as overlap syndrome or undifferentiated connective tissue disease, describes a set of connective tissue symptoms that overlap with other known connective tissue diseases. The imaging findings of mixed connective tissue disease include acroosteolysis, soft tissue calcification, myositis, and marrow edema. Erosions are uncommon in mixed connective tissue disease.

Reference: Manaster BJ, Roberts CC, Petersilge CA, et al. *Diagnostic Imaging: Musculoskeletal: Non-Traumatic Disease*. Philadelphia, PA: Amirsys; 2010;6:70.

17   Answer D.   Primary hand osteoarthritis is a peripheral arthropathy that involves the distal interphalangeal (DIP) joints, proximal interphalangeal (PIP) joints, and thumb carpometacarpal joints (CMC) with relative sparing of the metacarpophalangeal (MCP) joints. The soft tissue swelling associated with osteophytes around the DIP joint is called a Heberden node and around the PIP joint is called a Bouchard node. Nonuniform loss of cartilage results in bone hypertrophy manifesting as subchondral sclerosis and osteophyte development in the area of greatest loss of cartilage. The osteophytes of primary osteoarthritis must not be confused with either the new bone formation of psoriasis or the flared bone edges caused by psoriatic erosions.

Reference: Brower AC, Flemming DJ. *Arthritis in Black and White*. 3rd ed. Philadelphia, PA: Saunders; 2012:243–248.

18   Answer A.   The hallmarks of primary synovial osteochondromatosis are the numerable calcified and ossified nodules in the joint and synovium, with shallow, well-marginated erosions. The multiple, intracapsular nodules result in swelling, joint effusion, and secondary degenerative arthritis. The median age of presentation is in the sixth decade. There is a male predominance of nearly 2:1. The most common sites are the knee (70%) and the hip (20%). The condition is most frequently monoarticular, and the malignant risk of chondrosarcoma is rare (<5%). The main differential diagnosis is pigmented villonodular synovitis, which causes erosions similar to synovial osteochondromatosis without the calcifications.

Reference: Chew FS, Mulcahy H, Ha AS. *Musculoskeletal Imaging: A Teaching File*. 3rd ed. Philadelphia, PA: Lippincott Williams & Wilkins; 2012:233.

19   Answer B.   The patient presented has a history of multiple bowel surgeries and chronic abdominal and back pain, consistent with Crohn disease. Enteric arthritis can be seen in 10% to 15% of patients with inflammatory bowel disease. Typically, the joint involvement is similar to ankylosing spondylitis with sacroiliitis and syndesmophyte formation in the spine. Like ankylosing spondylitis, the sacroiliac joint involvement is usually bilateral and symmetric. It may be asymmetric at any time in the setting of inflammatory bowel disease. If there is asymmetric sacroiliac joint involvement, both sacroiliac joints are usually involved, as in the provided case. Psoriatic and reactive arthritis may initially have asymmetric sacroiliitis, but over time, this typically becomes bilaterally symmetric. Psoriatic and reactive arthritides, however, do not have syndesmophytes of the spine. Instead, they have bulky paravertebral ossifications, which extend vertically from the vertebral body. These are asymmetric with skip levels of uninvolved vertebral bodies. Septic arthritis of the sacroiliac joints is more commonly unilateral with sparing of the contralateral side.

Reference: Manaster BJ, Roberts CC, Petersilge CA, et al. *Diagnostic Imaging: Musculoskeletal: Non-Traumatic Disease*. Philadelphia, PA: Amirsys; 2010;1:88–93.

20a   **Answer D.**   Reactive arthritis was formerly known as Reiter syndrome. Classically, the syndrome is a combination of urethritis or cervicitis, conjunctivitis, and arthritis, which may present as asymmetric sacroiliac joint inflammation. Radiographically, reactive arthritis may present with normal bone density or periarticular osteopenia. Enthesopathy at tendon insertions is a prevalent finding, particularly at the Achilles insertion. The digits may have soft tissue swelling and periostitis. Sacroiliitis is usually asymmetric early but may become symmetric at any point in the disease. The spine demonstrates large, asymmetric, paravertebral ossifications.

References: Jacobson JA, Girish G, Jiang Y, et al. Radiographic evaluation of arthritis: inflammatory conditions. *Radiology*. 2008;248(2):378–389.
Manaster BJ, Roberts CC, Petersilge CA, et al. *Diagnostic Imaging: Musculoskeletal: Non-Traumatic Disease*. Philadelphia, PA: Amirsys; 2010;1:100–105.

20b   **Answer A.**   The cause is often unknown. There is a strong HLA-B27 association. It may be triggered by genitourinary tract infections, particularly by *Chlamydia trachomatis*. *Shigella, Salmonella, Yersinia*, and *Campylobacter* are known gastrointestinal infections, which may trigger the disease as well. Cultures of the joint fluid and synovium are negative, which is why the disease is coined reactive arthritis.

References: Jacobson JA, Girish G, Jiang Y, et al. Radiographic evaluation of arthritis: inflammatory conditions. *Radiology*. 2008;248(2):378–389.
Manaster BJ, Roberts CC, Petersilge CA, et al. *Diagnostic Imaging: Musculoskeletal: Non-Traumatic Disease*. Philadelphia, PA: Amirsys; 2010;1:100–105.

21   **Answer B.**   The sacral cartilage is thicker than the iliac cartilage; thus, early erosive changes of sacroiliitis are seen most commonly on the iliac side. The upper two-thirds of the sacroiliac joint is fibrous, and the inferior one-third of the joint is synovial; therefore, erosions occur in the inferior aspect of the joint. Many seronegative spondyloarthropathies involve the sacroiliac joints. In this case, the left sacroiliac joint is fused while the right sacroiliac joint demonstrates asymmetric widening, consistent with early ankylosing spondylitis. Over time, bilateral ankylosis will occur. In early sacroiliitis, erosions and cortical resorption around the joint lead to apparent joint space widening. Bone reparative changes in later stages of sacroiliitis result in subchondral sclerosis, joint space narrowing, and eventual ankylosis.

Reference: Brower AC, Flemming DJ. *Arthritis in Black and White*. 3rd ed. Philadelphia, PA: Saunders; 2012:226–230.

22   **Answer B.**   The image demonstrates muscle and soft tissue atrophy with soft tissue calcifications in the fascial planes of the proximal limbs. Early in the disease, manifestations of dermatomyositis include deep and superficial soft tissue edema in a symmetric and proximal distribution. MR images will show increased T2-weighted signal intensity. Later stages of disease involvement are characterized by muscle atrophy and fibrosis. Location and distribution may help differentiate this entity from other forms of autoimmune myopathy. Subcutaneous calcifications, similar to scleroderma, may be present. Articular abnormalities are uncommon but, when present, as in this case, are seen as uniform joint space loss with minimal bone hypertrophic changes. Bone scans may detect uptake of radionuclide in the soft tissues.

Reference: Brower AC, Flemming DJ. *Arthritis in Black and White*. 3rd ed. Philadelphia, PA: Saunders; 2012:354.

23 **Answer C.** Primary hemochromatosis is an inherited disorder that leads to massive iron deposition throughout the body. The initial presenting complaint of patients with hemochromatosis is joint pain, with as many as 50% of patients developing arthropathy. The predominant articular changes are those of a degenerative process, but the distribution is not that of primary osteoarthritis. The distribution of findings in hemochromatosis parallels that of the chronic degenerative form of calcium pyrophosphate dihydrate crystal deposition disease. Osteoporosis may be the only discriminating feature of hemochromatosis, which is not present in CPPD arthropathy. The clinical features suggest hemochromatosis as the underlying cause. The classic clinical triad is bronze skin, cirrhosis, and diabetes.

References: Askari AD, Muir WA, Rosner IA, et al. Arthritis of hemochromatosis. Clinical spectrum, relation to histocompatibility antigens, and effectiveness of early phlebotomy. *Am J Med*. 1983;75(6):957–965.
Brower AC, Flemming DJ. *Arthritis in Black and White*. 3rd ed. Philadelphia, PA: Saunders; 2012:335–338.

24 **Answer D.** The intervertebral joint is a combination of three joints consisting of the anterior column, disc, and the two facet joints of the posterior column supported by ligaments and muscle groups. As degenerative disc disease progresses, this degeneration stresses the facet joints and leads to facet arthropathy. The degenerative process of the facet may lead to ligamentum flavum hypertrophy and is an important component of lumbar stenosis. In combination with the ligamentum flavum hypertrophy, facet arthropathy, and facet ganglion cysts, the degeneration can result in a significant narrowing of the central canal, lateral recesses, and neural foramina.

References: Brower AC, Flemming DJ. *Arthritis in Black and White*. 3rd ed. Philadelphia, PA: Saunders; 2012:161–162.
Jinkins JR. Acquired degenerative changes of the intervertebral segments at and suprajacent to the lumbosacral junction. A radioanatomic analysis of the nondiscal structures of the spinal column and perispinal soft tissues. *Eur J Radiol*. 2004;50(2):134–158.
Malfair D, Beall DP. Imaging the degenerative diseases of the lumbar spine. *Magn Reson Imaging Clin N Am*. 2007;15(2):221–238.

25 **Answer B.** In this patient, the disc disease above the fusion has significantly progressed. The discs above and below the fusion undergo more stress due to restricted motion. Flexion and extension views are obtained to evaluate motion and disc height loss. The sequelae of degenerative disc disease are among the leading causes of functional incapacity. Degenerative disc disease is a multifactorial process that includes mechanical, traumatic, nutritional, and genetic factors that combine to variable degrees in different individuals. Disc disease is not an arthritis but combines with the facet arthropathy as spondylosis. The term disc degeneration includes disc desiccation, fibrosis, narrowing of the disc space, diffuse bulging of the annulus beyond the disc space, extensive fissuring, tears and mucinous degeneration of the annulus, endplate sclerosis, and osteophytes.

References: Brower AC, Flemming DJ. *Arthritis in Black and White*. 3rd ed. Philadelphia, PA: Saunders; 2012:161–162.
Modic MT, Ross JS. Lumbar degenerative disk disease. *Radiology*. 2007;245(1):43–61.

26 **Answer D.** Calcinosis circumscripta is dystrophic calcification, which may occur in either a localized or generalized pattern in the cutaneous and subcutaneous soft tissues. They are firm white dermal papules, plaques, or subcutaneous nodules that can ulcerate extruding a chalky white material. Calcinosis circumscripta can be seen following trauma, associated with connective tissue disorders (including polymyositis, dermatomyositis, and lupus) and inherited disorders such as Ehlers-Danlos syndrome. The calcifications may occur in bursa. Any type of metabolic calcification can potentially cause calcinosis circumscripta. Tumoral calcinosis is amorphous, cystic, and multilobulated calcification located in a periarticular distribution. The soft tissue masses in tumoral calcinosis do not erode or destroy adjacent bone. Calcific tendonitis is hydroxyapatite deposition within tendons and bursa. It may be asymptomatic or painful, but is usually self-limiting with resolution of imaging findings and symptoms.

Reference: Olsen KM, Chew FS. Tumoral calcinosis: pearls, polemics, and alternative possibilities. *Radiographics*. 2006:26(3):871–885.

27 **Answer B.**   The destruction of articular hyaline cartilage results in radiographic joint space narrowing. In osteoarthritis, the cartilage loss typically occurs in the weight-bearing portions of a joint. Additional findings of osteoarthritis include subchondral cyst formation and osteophytes. Osseous erosions are not a feature of conventional osteoarthritis, but central erosions are a feature of erosive osteoarthritis. In the hand and wrist, osteoarthritis typically involves the interphalangeal, the first carpometacarpal, and the scaphotrapeziotrapezoidal articulations.

Reference: Manaster BJ, May DA, Disler DG. *Musculoskeletal Imaging: The Requisites.* 4th ed. Philadelphia, PA: Mosby; 2013:263–270.

28 **Answer C.**   Diffuse idiopathic skeletal hyperostosis (DISH) is not a true arthropathy but a bone-forming diathesis. DISH is an enthesopathy that primarily ossifies ligaments and tendons. The flowing paraspinal osteophytes, which are characteristic of DISH, represent ossification of the longitudinal ligaments. DISH does not affect joint cartilage, articulating bone, or the disc spaces. DISH is most commonly observed in the thoracic spine and, unlike ankylosing spondylitis, it does not ossify Sharpey fibers. The ossification at the disc spaces bulges anteriorly. The diagnosis of DISH is made when this flowing ossification involves four or more contiguous vertebral bodies with their intervening disc spaces. In the cervical spine, DISH ossification may be so large that it causes dysphagia.

Reference: Taljanovic MS, Hunter TB, Wisneski RJ, et al. Imaging characteristics of diffuse idiopathic skeletal hyperostosis with an emphasis on acute spinal fractures: review. *AJR Am J Roentgenol.* 2009;193(3 Suppl):S10–S19.

29 **Answer B.**   The increased subchondral bone density in this patient is the result of bone hypertrophy triggered by the inflammation in osteoarthritis. The patellofemoral and medial femorotibial compartments are frequently involved.

Reference: Jacobson JA, Girish G, Jiang Y, et al. Radiographic evaluation of arthritis: inflammatory conditions. *Radiology.* 2008;248(2):378–389.

30a **Answer C.**   The radiographs demonstrate severe nonuniform joint space narrowing of the thumb carpometacarpal joint space with osteophyte formation. Subchondral sclerosis and subchondral cysts are present. These findings are consistent with osteoarthritis of the thumb carpometacarpal joint. Thumb carpometacarpal joint involvement in rheumatoid arthritis is uncommon. There are no erosions of the metacarpal heads or scaphoid in the provided images. Reactive arthritis most commonly involves the foot and calcaneus. The fingers can be involved, but the wrist and carpometacarpal joint involvement is uncommon. Hand and wrist involvement in ankylosing spondylitis is uncommon. Approximately 10% of ankylosing spondylitis patients have elbow, hand, and foot involvement.

References: Brower AC, Flemming DJ. *Arthritis in Black and White.* 3rd ed. Philadelphia, PA: Saunders; 2012:170–176, 220,241, 243–248.
Jacobson JA, Girish G, Jiang Y, et al. Radiographic evaluation of arthritis: inflammatory conditions. *Radiology.* 2008;248(2):378–389.

30b Answer A.   The excrescences noted arising from both the trapezium and the metacarpal are large osteophytes, seen in association with osteoarthritis. Enthesophytes, syndesmophytes, and erosions are not part of the constellation of findings noted in osteoarthritis.

References: Brower AC, Flemming DJ. *Arthritis in Black and White*. 3rd ed. Philadelphia, PA: Saunders; 2012:170–176, 220, 241, 243–248.
Jacobson JA, Girish G, Jiang Y, et al. Radiographic evaluation of arthritis: inflammatory conditions. *Radiology*. 2008;248(2):378–389.

31 Answer A.   The radiographs depict a case of erosive osteoarthritis. The differentiation of subchondral cysts from erosions can be difficult in the hand and wrist. Subchondral cysts form in the subchondral bone as a result of cartilage fissuring and extension of joint fluid into the underlying bone. Large subchondral cysts may be called geodes. The fluid mainly consists of hyaluronic acid, which is found in normal joint fluid. Erosions, on the other hand, destroy the bone cortex. In this case, the patient has findings of osteoarthritis that include peripheral, asymmetric joint involvement with asymmetric joint space loss, subchondral cysts, and osteophytosis. The patient also has central erosions, which have resulted in the gull wing appearance characteristic of erosive osteoarthritis.

Reference: Brower AC, Flemming DJ. *Arthritis in Black and White*. 3rd ed. Philadelphia, PA: Saunders; 2012:41–44.

32 Answer A.   One of the distinguishing features of psoriatic arthritis is bone proliferation. This can occur at erosions, across joints, along bone shafts, and at insertions of ligaments and tendons. Periostitis is bone proliferation along shafts of bone. Periostitis begins as fluffy mineralization and over time becomes solid new bone formation along the shaft of the bone. Bone proliferation is not a feature of the other answer choices but may be seen in reactive arthritis.

Reference: Brower AC, Flemming DJ. *Arthritis in Black and White*. 3rd ed. Philadelphia, PA: Saunders; 2012:200–205.

33 Answer C.   When there is symmetric uniform cartilage loss in the femoroacetabular joint, axial or superomedial migration of the femoral head occurs. Any disease process that uniformly destroys the cartilage in the hip will manifest as axial migration. Arthropathies that cause axial migration of the hip include rheumatoid arthritis, calcium pyrophosphate dihydrate crystal deposition disease, and ankylosing spondylitis. Acromegaly and ochronosis can also cause axial migration. Superolateral migration is seen in osteoarthritis. Medial migration is common in patients with primary osteoarthritis or in patients with posttraumatic osteoarthritis.

Reference: Brower AC, Flemming DJ. *Arthritis in Black and White*. 3rd ed. Philadelphia, PA: Saunders; 2012:93–102.

34 Answer B.   Juvenile idiopathic arthritis (JIA) is a constellation of diseases that manifest as a synovial inflammatory arthritis in children. JIA is classified on the basis of the number of joints involved, clinical symptoms, and serologic findings. The early radiographic findings of JIA are nonspecific. Early findings include soft tissue swelling, joint effusion, and osteopenia. Erosions are less common in JIA than in rheumatoid arthritis in adults due to the amount of cartilage at the epiphyses in children. In the cervical spine, ankylosis of synovial-lined apophyseal joints occurs at a young age. This leads to a decrease in size of the adjoining vertebral bodies, as well as a decrease in size of the corresponding disc spaces. This most commonly occurs at C2–C3, and the lower cervical spine is not involved without involvement of the superior cervical spine.

Radiography allows the accurate assessment of chronic changes of JIA, including growth disturbances, periostitis, and joint malalignment. Findings of active inflammation are best evaluated with ultrasound or MRI. US is sensitive for the detection of synovial proliferation and joint effusions. MRI may be utilized in JIA as it is a sensitive modality for detecting synovitis. Although sensitive for evaluating synovitis, MR is costly and time consuming and may require sedation for some pediatric patients. If there is suspected involvement of the temporomandibular or sacroiliac joints, MR is the best imaging tool due to the complexity of these joints.

References: Brower AC, Flemming DJ. *Arthritis in Black and White*. 3rd ed. Philadelphia, PA: Saunders; 2012: 357–369.

Sheybani EF, Khanna G, White AJ, et al. Imaging of juvenile idiopathic arthritis: a multimodality approach. *Radiographics*. 2013;33(5):1253–1273.

35 **Answer C.**   Knee arthroplasties have good-to-excellent results in 95% of patients with a 95% survival rate of the implant at 15 years, which is similar to that for hip prostheses. The total knee prosthesis hardware has femoral, tibial, and patellar radiopaque components and a spacer that is radiolucent. Some spacers have metallic markers, which help with visualization. In this case, a medial compartment prosthesis is seen with a spacer denoted by a metallic marker. The spacer is displaced toward the tibial eminence on the AP view and anteriorly and superiorly on the lateral view.

Aseptic loosening, periprosthetic fractures, and infection are complications of knee arthroplasty. Bone changes that may occur include periprosthetic lucency or lines, polyethylene wear, osteolysis, and change in prosthesis position. Focal nonprogressive radiolucent areas around the prosthesis components <2 mm in size are viewed as benign. Tibial component failure is more common than femoral component failure.

Reference: Taljanovic MS, Jones MD, Hunter TB, et al. Joint arthroplasties and prostheses. *Radiographics*. 2003;23(5):1295–1314.

36 **Answer A.**   Hallux rigidus is a condition characterized by loss of first metatarsophalangeal (MTP) joint motion due to degenerative arthritis. Osteophyte formation and osteoarthritis lead to dorsal impingement. The cause is a combination of acute trauma and repetitive microtrauma. Turf toe is an injury to the great toe plantar plate that is diagnosed by clinical exam and MRI. Morton syndrome is a condition where the second ray is significantly longer than the first, which may be shorter than normal. Altered weight bearing and mechanics in Morton syndrome predispose the patient to pain, dysfunction, and stress fractures. Hallux valgus deformity is an apex medial angulation of the great toe at the MTP joint. There is resultant soft tissue swelling and bony bunion formation. The altered foot mechanics can lead to early arthritis.

Reference: Karasick D, Wapner KL. Hallux rigidus deformity: radiologic assessment. *AJR Am J Roentgenol*. 1991;157(5):1029–1033.

37 **Answer D.**   The AP radiograph of the bilateral feet demonstrates diffuse osteopenia. There is uniform joint space narrowing of the second through fifth metatarsophalangeal joints. There are large erosions of the bilateral fifth metatarsal heads. Erosions are also seen in the heads of the second, third, and fourth metatarsals. These findings are consistent with rheumatoid arthritis. Nonerosive osteoarthritis would manifest as joint space narrowing but no erosive changes. Psoriatic arthritis would produce "pencil-in-cup" erosions; in the foot, interphalangeal joint space involvement is more common than metatarsophalangeal joint space involvement. Ankylosing spondylitis is an axial arthropathy that typically involves the spine. Gout also produces erosions, but they are usually extra-articular and in the foot predominantly involve the great toe metatarsophalangeal joint.

Reference: Brower AC, Flemming DJ. *Arthritis in Black and White*. 3rd ed. Philadelphia, PA: Saunders; 2012:171–177.

38 Answer A.   The earliest radiographic changes of rheumatoid arthritis in the hand and wrist are symmetric periarticular soft tissue swelling around the involved joints with juxta-articular osteoporosis. Erosions may precede joint space loss. As the disease progresses, there is uniform joint space loss. Late in the disease, soft tissue swelling subsides, the osteoporosis becomes diffuse, and the erosions enlarge. Metacarpophalangeal joint subluxation is also a late finding. There may be ulnar subluxation of the carpus as well.

Reference: Brower AC, Flemming DJ. *Arthritis in Black and White*. 3rd ed. Philadelphia, PA: Saunders; 2012:171–177.

39 Answer B.   The sagittal CT image shows severe L3–L4 disc space narrowing with vacuum disc phenomenon. Anterior osteophytes are noted at multiple levels. At L3–L4, there is endplate eburnation. Discitis–osteomyelitis is unlikely in this case since the endplates are preserved. In addition, vacuum phenomenon argues against discitis–osteomyelitis. Thin flowing syndesmophytes would be expected in ankylosing spondylitis with the "bamboo spine" as a late manifestation. In diffuse idiopathic skeletal hyperostosis (DISH), the intervertebral disc spaces are usually preserved, and there are bulky ossifications anterior to the vertebral body.

Reference: Brower AC, Flemming DJ. *Arthritis in Black and White*. 3rd ed. Philadelphia, PA: Saunders; 2012:155–162.

40 Answer B.   A change in the position of an implant is the most specific sign for arthroplasty loosening. This change may be seen as subsidence of a component into the underlying bone or tilting of a component. Positional change may be subtle and only detected when comparison is made with prior exams. A cemented component may show slight lucency at the interface between bone and cement, but is not considered by most to be a radiographic manifestation of loosening until it is >2 mm and surrounds the majority of the component. The presence of an implant alters the stress loading on the native bone. This alteration may lead to a reduction in bone mass and a loss of bone density, termed stress shielding. It characteristically occurs in the proximal femoral shaft in the setting of a total hip arthroplasty. Polyethylene wear is thinning of the component in the weight-bearing region as compared to other areas of the liner.

References: Fritz J, Lurie B, Miller TT. Imaging of hip arthroplasty. *Semin Musculoskelet Radiol*. 2013;17(3):316–327.
Keogh CF, Munk PL, Gee R, et al. Imaging of the painful hip arthroplasty. *AJR Am J Roentgenol*. 2003;180(1):115–120.

1 Which of the following is the most common tumor complication associated with the disorder depicted by the radiograph?

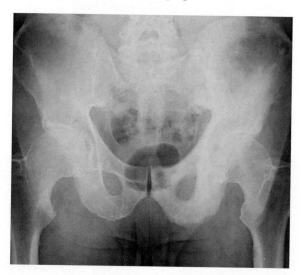

A. Lymphoma
B. Sarcoma
C. Giant cell tumor
D. Enchondroma

2 Which disease is characterized by periarticular tendinous thickening, thickened synovium, and large erosions?

A. Rheumatoid arthritis
B. Hemophilic arthropathy
C. Amyloidosis
D. Gout

3 Which of the following diseases most likely manifests as a diffuse bony sclerosis?

A. Mastocytosis
B. Osteomalacia
C. Multiple myeloma
D. Vitamin C deficiency

4 A 57-year-old female presents with lower extremity pain. Based on the images below, which of the following is the next most appropriate study?

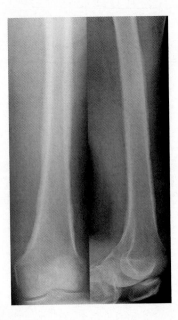

    A. Cervical spine radiograph
    B. Lumbar spine MRI
    C. Abdomen and pelvis CT
    D. Chest radiograph

5 Sagittal MR images of the cervical spine of a 16-month-old patient demonstrate which of the following osseous findings?

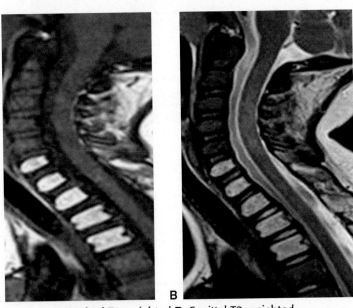

A. Sagittal T1 weighted **B.** Sagittal T2 weighted

    A. Leukemic infiltration
    B. Postradiation changes
    C. Rickets
    D. Red marrow conversion

6 Which of the following best describes the imaging appearance of sarcoidosis in the hand?

A. Soft tissue swelling and periarticular erosions with overhanging edges
B. Periarticular osteoporosis and marginal erosions
C. Lace-like trabecular pattern and cortical erosions
D. Joint space narrowing and subluxations

7a The radiograph of the pelvis below demonstrates the imaging findings characteristic of what diagnosis?

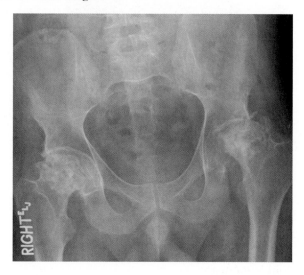

A. Slipped capital femoral epiphysis
B. Osteonecrosis
C. Trauma
D. Osteoarthrosis

7b The MR images below depict what sign that is typically associated with osteonecrosis of the hip?

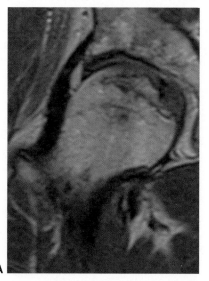 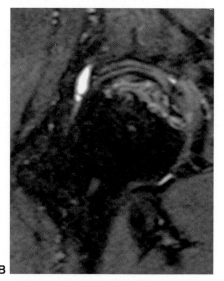

A. Coronal proton density **B.** Coronal T2 weighted fat saturated

A. Crescent sign
B. Joint effusion sign
C. Increased T2 cortex signal sign
D. Double-line sign

8a The following radiograph demonstrates the blade of grass sign, characteristic of which of the following pathologies?

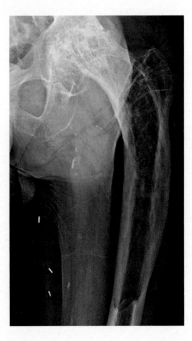

A. Radiation osteonecrosis
B. Paget disease
C. Acute myeloid leukemia
D. Sarcoidosis

8b Which of the following is the best definition for the term "blade of grass"?

A. Site of sarcomatous degeneration
B. Site of pathologic fracture
C. Thickened cortex in long bones
D. Sharp demarcation in long bones between lesion and normal bone

9 A 10-year-old male presents with thickening of the skin of the face. Radiographs of the forearm demonstrate periosteal reaction of the distal radial and ulnar metaphyses. These findings are most characteristic of which of the following diseases?

A. Primary hypertrophic osteoarthropathy
B. Rickets
C. Juvenile idiopathic arthritis
D. Fluorosis

ANSWERS AND EXPLANATIONS

1 **Answer B.** Neoplastic complications associated with Paget disease are relatively rare and have been reported to occur in <1% of cases with limited skeletal involvement and up to 5% to 10% of cases with widespread skeletal involvement. Sarcomatous transformation is the most common manifestation of a neoplastic complication. The most common type of sarcomatous transformation is osteosarcoma. Imaging findings that would be concerning for sarcomatous transformation include aggressive osteolysis, cortical destruction, and an associated soft tissue mass.

References: Smith SE, Murphey MD, Motamedi K, et al. From the archives of the AFIP. Radiologic spectrum of Paget disease of bone and its complications with pathologic correlation. *Radiographics.* 2002;22:1191–1216.

Theodorou DJ, Theodorou SJ, Kakitsubata Y. Imaging of Paget disease of bone and its musculoskeletal complications: review. *AJR Am J Roentgenol.* 2011;196:S64–S75.

2 **Answer C.** Amyloidosis is a multisystem disorder caused by abnormal extracellular deposition of protein and protein derivatives. Amyloid arthropathy is an erosive and destructive arthropathy. Periarticular tendon thickening, due to amyloid infiltration, joint effusions, bursitis, capsular thickening, thickened synovium, and large erosions are musculoskeletal characteristics of this disease. On MR imaging, the tendons, capsule, and synovium will be low in signal intensity on all sequences. Erosions are typically filled with low signal intensity material. Muscular infiltration may also occur and cause hypertrophy, chronic pain, and weakness, which preferentially involve the shoulder girdle. Patients usually appear to have well-developed shoulder musculature, which is asymmetric to the patient's other musculature, and is termed the shoulder pad sign. In contradistinction to amyloid arthropathy, erosions in rheumatoid arthritis contain high signal intensity material on fluid-sensitive sequences, and rheumatoid nodules are typically subcutaneous and are often adjacent to a bony prominence such as the olecranon. In hemophilic arthropathy, chronic hemosiderin deposition results in blooming artifact on gradient echo imaging. Gout is characterized by soft tissue tophi, which may contain calcifications, and juxta-articular erosions with overhanging margins.

References: Georgiades CS, Neyman EG, Barish MA, et al. Amyloidosis: review and CT manifestations. *Radiographics.* 2004;24:405–416.

Manaster BJ, Roberts CC, Petersilge CA, et al. *Diagnostic Imaging: Musculoskeletal: Non-Traumatic Disease.* Manitoba, Canada: Amirsys; 2010:1:124–129.

3 **Answer A.** Bone involvement in mastocytosis may be lytic, sclerotic, or a mixed process due to the release of histamine and prostaglandins. Diffuse involvement tends to be more common, but the involvement of the axial skeleton is predominant. Usually, the radiographic appearance is that of sclerosis involving primarily the axial skeleton and the ends of long bones. In some patients, there is generalized osteoporosis with a risk for pathologic fractures. Imaging is helpful to establish the extent of the disease. Osteomalacia causes abnormal bone mineralization and may result in Looser zones (fractures) in adults. Multiple myeloma is characterized by widespread, osseous lytic lesions. Vitamin C deficiency and scurvy result in abnormal epiphyseal and metaphyseal development such as metaphyseal cupping and dense metaphyseal lines in infants and children. Musculoskeletal manifestations of scurvy in adults include severe joint pain and hemarthrosis.

Reference: Fritz J, Fishman EK, Carrino JA, et al. Advanced imaging of skeletal manifestations of systemic mastocytosis. *Skeletal Radiol.* 2012;41(8):887–897.

4   **Answer D.**   The images depict diffuse periosteal reaction without an underlying osseous abnormality, consistent with hypertrophic osteoarthropathy. Hypertrophic osteoarthropathy may be primary in etiology in 3% to 5% of cases, while 95% to 97% of cases are the result of a secondary etiology. 90% of secondary hypertrophic osteoarthropathy cases are the result of malignancy, with non–small cell lung cancer being the most common cause. Therefore, imaging of the chest is the most appropriate next study. In this case, imaging of the chest revealed a large primary lung malignancy. The most common locations for diffuse periosteal reaction to be noted are the tibia and fibula followed by the radius and ulna. In this case, the findings were also present in the tibia and fibula, but were more obvious in the femur.

Reference: Manaster BJ, Roberts CC, Petersilge CA, et al. *Diagnostic Imaging: Musculoskeletal: Non-Traumatic Disease*. Manitoba, Canada: Amirsys; 2010:1:162–167.

5   **Answer B.**   The sagittal MR images show homogeneously hyperintense T1- and T2-weighted signal in five consecutive vertebral bodies. This sharp demarcation of fatty marrow is secondary to a radiation port for the treatment of neuroblastoma. Bone marrow changes induced by therapeutic radiation have a predictable evolution because of the direct effects on the cellular components of bone as well as the indirect effects of vascular injury. The T1-weighted signal is increased in the involved bone due to replacement of the hematopoietic marrow with fat, which may be seen 3 months after initiation of therapy and remain indefinitely. Over time, marrow fibrosis can develop; fibrosis should have low T1-weighted and T2-weighted signal intensities. Other effects of radiation therapy include osteonecrosis, insufficiency fractures, and radiation-induced neoplasms. In the growing skeleton, radiation may cause bone growth cessation, fractures (i.e., slipped capital epiphysis), and scoliosis.

Reference: Mitchell MJ, Logan PM. Radiation-induced changes in bone. *Radiographics*. 1998;18:1125–1136.

6   **Answer C.**   The characteristic lace-like or honeycomb appearance is caused by the presence of multiple granulomatous lesions in the bones of the hands or feet. Granulomas within or next to the bone may erode the cortex or cause lytic lesions with nonaggressive features within the medullary cavity. Sarcoidosis affects the bones in 10% of patients with pulmonary findings, but sarcoidosis more often causes transient migratory polyarticular arthralgias without radiographic changes. Additional skeletal findings include joint abnormalities and marrow infiltration of small and large bones. Long bone and axial skeletal involvement may be occult on conventional radiography, but the MRI appearance may resemble that of osseous metastases.

Reference: Moore SL, Teirstein AE. Musculoskeletal sarcoidosis: spectrum of appearances at MR imaging. *Radiographics*. 2003;23:1389–1399.

7a   **Answer B.**   Osteonecrosis is also known as ischemic necrosis, aseptic necrosis, and avascular necrosis. It results in necrosis of the cellular elements of bone secondary to ischemia. This ischemia may be posttraumatic in nature, resulting in a disrupted blood supply. Alternatively, it may be the result of corticosteroid use, which causes enlargement of the intramedullary fat cells and consequently leads to increased intramedullary pressure and inhibition of blood flow. Patchy sclerosis of the femoral head is an early radiographic finding. Late radiographic findings in the hip include femoral head irregularity and fragmentation, collapse of the femoral head articular surface, and secondary osteoarthrosis.

References: Manaster BJ, May DA, Disler DG. *Musculoskeletal Imaging: The Requisites*. 4th ed. Philadelphia, PA: Saunders; 2013:346–350.
Manaster BJ, Roberts CC, Petersilge CA, et al. *Diagnostic Imaging: Musculoskeletal: Non-Traumatic Disease*. Manitoba, Canada: Amirsys; 2010:10:8–13.

7b Answer D.   On MR imaging, the double-line sign is classically seen in association with osteonecrosis. This finding is depicted by a low signal intensity line along the periphery of the infarct and a brighter signal line at the interface with the infarcted bone. The crescent sign is a radiographic finding in osteonecrosis indicating a subchondral fracture.

References: Manaster BJ, May DA, Disler DG. *Musculoskeletal Imaging: The Requisites.* 4th ed. Philadelphia, PA: Saunders; 2013:346–350.
Manaster BJ, Roberts CC, Petersilge CA, et al. *Diagnostic Imaging: Musculoskeletal: Non-Traumatic Disease.* Manitoba, Canada: Amirsys; 2010:10:8–13.

8a Answer B.   The blade of grass sign or flame sign represents a wedge or V-shaped area of radiolucency typically located in the diaphysis of a long bone. The sign is characteristic of the lytic phase of Paget disease. Paget disease is typified by an increase in osteoclast-mediated bone resorption, which is accompanied by a compensatory increase in bone formation. There are three phases to Paget disease: lytic, sclerotic, and mixed. Most often, affected bones demonstrate a coarsened trabecular pattern and cortical thickening that encroaches on the medullary cavity. The most commonly affected bones are the pelvis, lumbar spine, femur, tibia, and skull. Paget disease is polyostotic in most cases but may be monostotic in 10% to 35% of cases.

References: Manaster BJ, Roberts CC, Petersilge CA, et al. *Diagnostic Imaging. Musculoskeletal: Non-Traumatic Disease.* Manitoba, Canada: Amirsys; 2010:2:184–186.
Wittenberg K. The blade of grass sign. *Radiology.* 2001;221:199–200.

8b Answer D.   The blade of grass sign is the demarcation between pagetoid bone and normal bone.

References: Manaster BJ, Roberts CC, Petersilge CA, et al. *Diagnostic Imaging. Musculoskeletal: Non-Traumatic Disease.* Manitoba, Canada: Amirsys; 2010:2:184–186.
Wittenberg K. The blade of grass sign. *Radiology.* 2001;221:199–200.

9 Answer A.   Primary hypertrophic osteoarthropathy, also known as pachydermoperiostosis, is a self-limited, autosomal dominant disease characterized by generalized and symmetric periosteal reaction with marked thickening of the skin of the extremities, face, and scalp. This disease is not associated with a secondary cause, such as lung disease. Most commonly, children or young adult males are affected with bone and joint pain. The pain typically decreases or resolves in adulthood. The periosteal reaction primarily involves the distal ends of the radius, ulna, tibia, and fibula.

References: Manaster BJ, Roberts CC, Petersilge CA, et al. *Diagnostic Imaging: Musculoskeletal: Non-Traumatic Disease.* Manitoba, Canada: Amirsys; 2010:164–167.
Rana RS, Wu JS, Eisenberg RL. Periosteal reaction. *AJR Am J Roentgenol.* 2009;193(4): W259–W272.